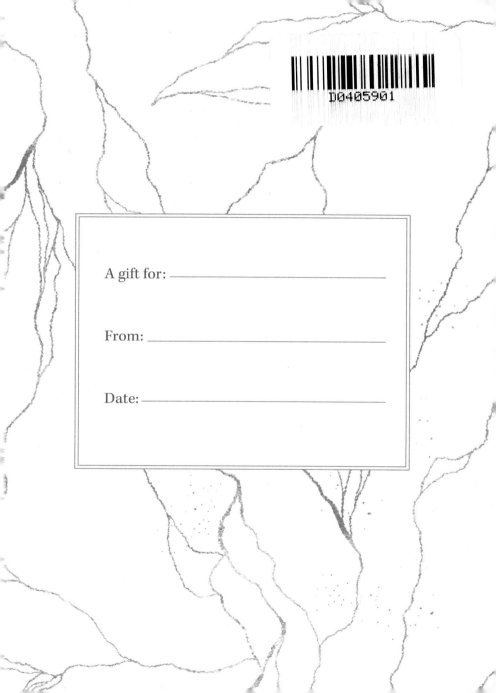

A gift for: _____

From: _____

Date: _____

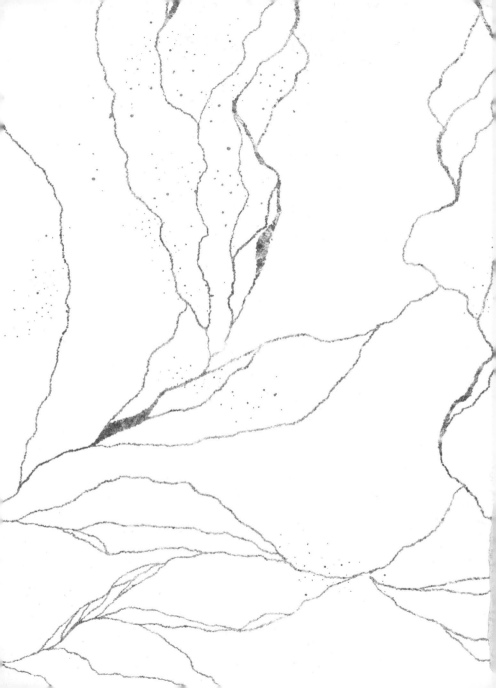

GLOW

90 DAYS TO CREATE YOUR
VIBRANT LIFE FROM WITHIN

DR. STACIE STEPHENSON

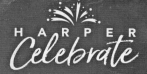

The information in this book has been carefully researched by the author and is intended to be a source of information only. Readers are urged to consult with their physicians or other professional advisors to address specific medical or other issues. The author and the publisher assume no responsibility for any injuries suffered or damages incurred during or as a result of the use or application of the information contained herein.

Glow

Published by Harper Celebrate, an imprint of HarperCollins Focus LLC.

Any internet addresses (websites, blogs, etc.) in this book are offered as a resource. They are not intended in any way to be or imply an endorsement by HarperCollins Focus LLC, nor does HarperCollins Focus LLC vouch for the content of these sites for the life of this book.

ISBN 978-1-4002-4014-2 (audiobook)
ISBN 978-1-4002-4015-9 (epub)
ISBN 978-1-4002-4013-5 (HC)

Printed in India

23 24 25 26 27 REP 5 4 3 2 1

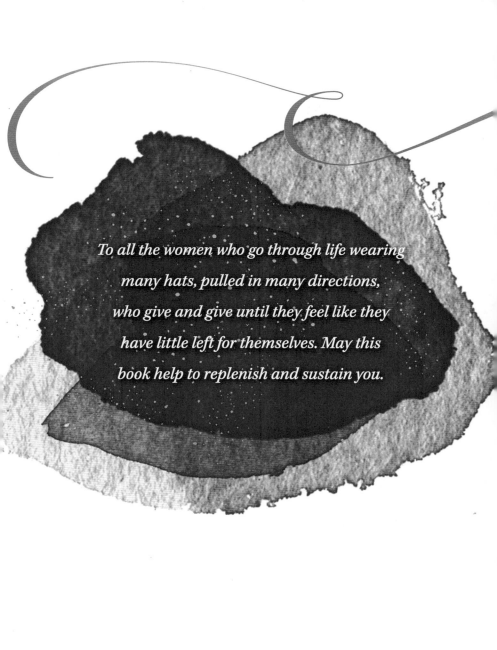

*To all the women who go through life wearing
many hats, pulled in many directions,
who give and give until they feel like they
have little left for themselves. May this
book help to replenish and sustain you.*

CONTENTS

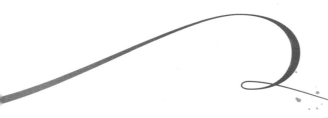

I reserve a sacred fifteen- to thirty-minute block of time at the beginning and end of every day. No matter how busy I get, whether I'm home or traveling, I prioritize these moments when I don't have any obligations and can sit all by myself, resting, reflecting, and setting my intentions for the day ahead or settling into a restful evening. This daily practice has been one of the most powerful and influential things I do to keep myself feeling mentally centered, physically healthy, emotionally balanced, socially connected, spiritually calm, and focused on my goals.

This book offers you the opportunity to hold a similar space for yourself each day. It contains ninety days of morning and evening meditations, intentions, inspirations, and motivational guidance for living a more vibrant life. These are things for you to contemplate and carry with you. These morning and evening thoughts are based on what I have found to be the most fruitful and productive things to think about during the quiet times I gift myself. Every entry is embedded with inspiration, motivation, and information to help you live a more full, satisfying, and glowing life. My hope is that you will find them energizing or relaxing as needed, and that they will help to improve and brighten the overall quality of your days.

Using the acronym VIBRANT, I've structured this book so that each day of the week has a theme:

V: Mondays are about Voice. Your voice includes how you talk to yourself as well as how you express your thoughts, feelings, and desires to the world around you. On Voice days, you will work on achieving a new level of self-awareness and courage to step into your life and make it what *you* want it to be, unburdened by the expectations of others. You'll examine the ways you talk— your negative and positive self-talk, how you articulate your thoughts, and how you can be a voice in support of others. Let the worries of potential judgments from others take a back seat, and learn how to use your unique voice to express exactly what you need to say.

I: Tuesdays are about Intuition. Intuition is your sense of inner knowing. We all have it, but sometimes that still, small whisper is hard to hear. And yet it is always talking to us, in the form of thoughts, feelings, hunches, and even physical symptoms, as our bodies give us constant feedback about what we're doing and whether it's good for us. On Intuition days, we'll work on honing this very special skill so you can build trust and confidence in your own inner sense of what is right, what is good, what is safe, and what is a warning. You'll learn how to do this physically as well as mentally and emotionally, as you focus inward, turning down the volume of your thoughts and the noisy world so you can hear what your intuition is trying to tell you.

B: Wednesdays are about Balance. The demands of daily life can often pull you in countless directions and away from your balanced center. Whether it's work-life balance, self-other balance, physical- and mental-energy balance, or any other kind of balancing act you're attempting, you'll get support midweek on these days. We'll cover strategies, tips, and techniques for exploring where imbalances exist, dialing back habits that aren't helping you, and establishing exercises and routines that lead to feeling better and accomplishing more. We'll also get into the wonders of the Vibrant Triad, a system I developed that can help you to achieve balance in the three foundational areas that largely determine health and wellness: what you eat, how you move, and how you connect with others.

R: Thursdays are about Rejuvenation. So much to do! It's easy to overextend, overexercise, overwork, overeat, and overdeplete, but on Rejuvenation days you're going to learn how to slow down and get the restoration you need to get back to your optimal state of being. With guidance for all kinds of regenerative strategies—like digital detoxes, healing baths, better sleep hygiene, morning routines that work, and physical habits to help your body regenerate for a more energetic, youthful you—you'll explore how to get back to feeling your best, especially during times of stress. Your nervous system is hardwired to gear up when you need it, but that can only happen if you also regularly decompress and recover.

A: Fridays are about Abundance. Abundance has to do with resources: physical, emotional, and spiritual. Many of us feel compelled to give endlessly and end up feeling empty because we neglect our own needs. To focus on abundance is to bring enough of the things you need into your life: love, support, meaningful relationships, connection with nature, fulfilling work, and you-time. When you have enough abundance in your life, when it overflows and fills you with gratitude, sharing with others will feel joyful and fulfilling. On Abundance days, we'll work on how you can explore and discover where you are most rich, and then, how giving and sharing your resources, time, or talents can actually increase abundance, lower stress, and infuse you with a deep sense of gratitude for the gifts in your life.

N: Saturdays are about Nurturing. An essential part of human connection is nurturing, and we can all probably get a little better at giving and receiving the gift of nurturing. Nurturing leads to growth, advancement, flourishing, and strengthened relationships, and we can gift it not just to our children but also to partners, parents, friends, coworkers, pets, and communities. On Nurturing days, we'll explore the many ways you can care for the people who populate your life through teaching, supporting, sharing passions, bonding physically and emotionally, and creating meaningful connections. And of course, I'll remind you how important it is to nurture yourself with all the love, care, and attention you offer to others.

T: Sundays are about Thoughtfulness. Focusing on others will infuse your Sundays with kindness and consideration, generosity, and the deep spiritual joy that comes from sending your energy outward to others. Sometimes I'll cue you to try meditation or prayer. Sometimes I'll suggest you focus on those who really need your attention, and sometimes I'll encourage you to explore the treasures you hold deep within—treasures you could offer to others. Thoughtful giving is the best remedy for stress or sadness because it takes you outside of yourself. On Thoughtfulness days, you can explore both your deep inner life and the ways you can best express your most open-handed and open-hearted impulses as you practice more intentional thoughtfulness.

In addition to these daily focal points, each week has a theme to help you explore this VIBRANT wisdom in the essential core areas of your life. Throughout the book, you'll also find forty mantras you can repeat to yourself throughout the day to stay focused and motivated. Several of the entries invite you to explore written exercises, so it is a good idea to keep a notebook or journal handy as you move through your journey toward a more vibrant tomorrow.

This is how you fill your own cup so you'll be better equipped to care for others, from family and friends to community and beyond. I've always believed that the small things we do over time accumulate to create life-changing shifts personally, locally, and globally. Wherever you are in your journey, this book is designed to meet you there and move you forward, one step at a time, for a ripple effect that could result in a kinder, healthier, smarter, more luminous and vibrant world.

It is my sincere hope that you will benefit in profound ways from these sacred moments alone with yourself and *Glow*. As you are practicing using your voice more purposefully, listening to your intuition, working on balance, exploring rejuvenation, increasing abundance in the areas that matter most, nurturing others, and living a more thoughtful life, you will feel yourself gradually becoming the benevolent master of your own body, mind, emotions, and spirit. You are worth this time, so I hope you will commit to using it for your growth. It's only a few minutes every morning and evening. You deserve that, and more. Now, get ready to experience what it really means to live, give, and glow vibrantly.

Dr. Stacie Stephenson

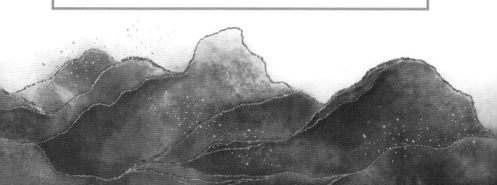

WEEK ONE:

Start with Self-Care

Being solitary is being alone well: being alone luxuriously immersed in doings of your own choice, aware of the fullness of your own presence rather than of the absence of others.

ALICE KOLLER

Voice:

HOW DO YOU TALK TO YOURSELF?

How you talk to yourself is a reflection of how you value yourself, and it matters. Does your self-talk reflect confidence and compassion or disrespect and insecurity? Today, see if you can tune in to the voice in your head. Without judging, simply *notice* what it's saying. When you wake up and look in the mirror, where do your thoughts go? If you make a mistake at work, does your inner voice default to berating you or to lifting you up and helping you to make it right and move on? See if you can notice patterns: When are you hard on yourself, and when are you self-supportive? When you notice a negative pattern, try reframing by asking yourself: *Would I say this to a friend in my position?* Try treating yourself with the same compassion you'd offer to that friend.

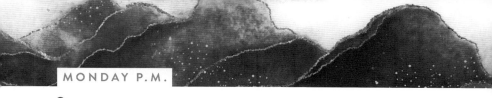

Voice:

STOP SPEAKING, AND LISTEN

After talking all day, out loud and in your own head, it can be difficult to turn off that voice when it's time to wind down for sleep. But just like your body, your voice needs to recover. It has worked hard for hours on end communicating with the external world. This evening, spend just ten minutes in intentional silence, and allow your physical voice to rest. This will give you the space you need to listen to your quiet inner voice—this is your internal communication system, and its messages are just for you. Listen to what it tells you that you need as you begin this week focused on self-care, and reassure yourself that whatever your internal voice asks for, you can provide.

Intuition:

DISCOVER YOUR TRUE NATURE

Intuition is quiet. The world is loud. Tapping into your inner sense of knowing can be challenging, but with practice, you can learn more about yourself. Today, pay attention to cues from your intuition. Are there times when you "have a feeling" about someone or have the thought that you should or shouldn't do something for an unknown reason? Are there moments when you think: *This is bad for me* or *This would be good for me*? Marvel at the complexity of your brain and body as it takes in external cues you don't consciously notice and translates them into information you can actually tune in to and use. Think about noticing these intuitive moments more often so they can guide you in how to better care for yourself and live according to your true nature. Try writing down what happens when you check in with your intuition throughout the day. What is it telling you?

Intuition:
YOU ALREADY KNOW WHAT YOU NEED

Let's revisit that list of intuitive moments you kept throughout the day. How well did you heed the call of your intuition? Evaluate when you felt a clear message coming in, and when your inner hesitation or external noise clouded the message. In moments when you did clearly hear your intuition, did you allow that signal to inform your actions? As you wind down tonight, see if you can get very quiet and let your intuition rise. Turn inward and feel what your intuition has to tell you about yourself and what you need. Do you need to give yourself some kind words? Some physical care, like eating better or moving more? Do you need to reach out to friends more often or rekindle romance in your life? Whatever it is, let your intuition guide you toward what you need most right now. When you are quiet, you'll get the most information.

Balance:

GIVE YOURSELF ONE FULL HOUR

It seems everybody is talking about self-care lately, but what does that mean, exactly? Self-care is a way to give yourself what you really need, whether that's rest, exercise, a good meal, or just some peace and quiet. To me, self-care is an essential part of balance, especially for anyone who spends a lot of time caring for others: partners, children, parents, friends, even pets. It's especially important for new parents and care-givers, who tend to give far more than they get back. Nobody knows what you really need more than *you* do—trust that you know yourself that well. Today, try to spend one full hour caring for your own needs in a way that will bring you back to center. That may sound like a lot, but this is an investment in your peace of mind. Prepare and enjoy nourishing food. Go for a walk. Call your favorite person. Read for pleasure. Or just take a nap. Even if you have to break up that hour into three or four sessions, let that time be just for you. I guarantee you'll feel more balanced, and that's good for your overall health.

Balance:
SELF VERSUS OTHER

This evening, consider how well you balanced "self" and "other" today. If you are used to giving most of your time and energy to others, it can be difficult to make a time commitment to self-care. Even if you gave yourself just a few minutes, that's a win. But where *did* most of your giving go today? Are there things you feel, in retrospect, got too much of your attention, and other things that didn't get enough? This evening, think about those areas that are important to you (not to anybody else, necessarily) that you wish you could spend more time on. Is there something you love to do, but you often prioritize other things ahead of it? Think about how you might allot your time tomorrow a bit differently, in a way that would be more personally fulfilling. I'm not talking about big changes. Small, gradual shifts toward giving yourself a little more time for your own needs and interests can feel both doable and deeply satisfying.

Rejuvenation:
EASE THE EFFECTS OF STRESS

With every passing year of life, the body changes in noticeable ways. You may not appreciate all of these changes, but they are physical signs that you are growing in wisdom and experience. Even so, rejuvenation of many of the body's systems is possible. You can't stop aging completely, but you can definitely slow the effects and even reverse those aspects of it that have been accelerated due to lifestyle factors. Stress ages the body, inside and out, so one of the most profound—and simple— ways to rejuvenate the body is through stress reduction. Deep breathing can reverse the stress response in just a few minutes. Today, take five minutes during your morning routine to sit in a quiet place undisturbed and breathe slowly and deeply. Make a mental note of what parts of your body feel like they're in need of extra care. Focus on letting your breath relax those parts of your body.

Rejuvenation:
EVENING EXFOLIATION

One of the most soothing ways to rejuvenate the body is with skin care. To help dull skin look and feel more radiant, add exfoliation to your evening routine. This simple step increases cell turnover and restores your skin's natural glow. You don't have to buy a fancy product. You can use your regular cleanser along with an exfoliating brush, sponge, or pad with texture. Use a light hand to stimulate circulation and remove dead skin cells without pulling on or scrubbing delicate facial skin. To reduce flaking and crepey skin on arms, legs, hands, and feet, you can get a little more aggressive with a dry-skin brush or a homemade scrub. Mix olive or almond oil and sugar to make a thick paste, and use it as a body scrub. (This is one of the few really good uses for sugar!) Rub it in—massaging your limbs, hands, and feet—then shower it off. Not only can consistent exfoliation really improve your skin's tone, resilience, moisture, and youthfulness, but it's a nice way to de-stress.

Abundance: ENHANCE
YOUR LIFE WITH GOOD HEALTH

It's often said that if you don't have your health, you don't have anything. That's not true, of course. Many people with ailing health are rich in family, friends, love, passion, curiosity, intellect, and more. I do believe, however, that health can *enhance* life: not just the enjoyment of it but the opportunities within it. That's why, to me, abundance starts with health. Glowing, vibrant health provides more energy, a sharper mind, a more comfortable body, and the opportunity to do more with your gifts. But to accumulate health abundance, you have to commit to taking care of your health in a world where vibrant health can feel elusive. We often think of physical discomforts as things we have to push through in order to get things done. Likewise, it's easy to take good health for granted or to notice it only when you begin to lose it. Instead, begin today by tuning in to your physical body to feel and assess your own health state. *Notice* how you feel: What ailments can you modulate and reduce rather than ignore, and what robust aspects of your health can you celebrate with gratitude? This is the very first step in what could become a fascinating and adventure-filled journey to health abundance and optimization.

Abundance: TONIGHT'S REST CREATES TOMORROW'S ENERGY

How do you grow in health abundance? One foundational way is to get consistent, high-quality sleep, which we'll talk about in more detail later on. A lack of good sleep can undermine the work you're pouring into physical and mental self-care, but a good long sleep of seven to nine hours can make all your good-health efforts feel easier. It can also reduce many symptoms of and triggers for chronic disease. You can eat perfectly and exercise daily, but if you aren't getting good sleep, you could still be breaking down your health. Tonight, see if you can go to bed thirty to sixty minutes earlier than usual. Turn off all the lights and devices, close your eyes, and imagine yourself glowing with vibrant health, and an inner sense of peace and calm, effortlessly relaxing your entire body and easily quieting your mind as sleep replenishes you. Let yourself drift off with this image of health abundance in your mind.

Nurturing:
GO EASY ON YOURSELF

While there is great joy to be found in caring for the people who populate your life, you might spend so much time nurturing others that you often forget to nurture yourself. But you need to protect your inner resources in order to support your loved ones in meaningful ways. How do you truly, deeply nurture yourself? There are some obvious ways (rest, quiet time, doing an activity that you love), but at the very foundation of self-nurturing is something that's not so easy to do: self-acceptance. Are you as forgiving of your own faults as you are of the faults of others? Today, try to exercise compassion for yourself, flaws and all. Even if it feels difficult, practice treating yourself with love, compassion, and forgiveness. You are only human, after all.

Nurturing:
SAY IT OUT LOUD

This evening, make a list of five things you love about yourself and five things you don't love so much. Be honest with yourself, not about what others might see as your short-comings but what *you see as your own faults*. Then, read your lists out loud.

Before everything on your first list, say: "I love that I . . ."

After everything on your second list, say: ". . . but I love who I am, I embrace my true nature, and I let go of the anxiety that comes from the false belief that I'm not enough."

For example:

"I love that I am creative."

And (this is harder than you might think, but do it anyway—out loud!): "I'm not self-confident, but I love who I am, I embrace my true nature, and I let go of the anxiety that comes from the false belief that I'm not enough."

Thoughtfulness: BECOME AN OBSERVER OF YOUR THOUGHTS

What does *thoughtfulness* mean to you? You may define it as thinking of others. That is part of thoughtfulness, but another part is to become more deliberate about and conscious of your own thought processes. Have you ever stopped to notice your thoughts, not from the inside as the person thinking them, but from the outside, as an observer? This is an ancient meditative practice that can bring perspective and calm when experiencing thoughts that may seem anxious or frenetic. Here's how to give it a try: Sit quietly and take a few deep breaths, close your eyes, then imagine watching your thoughts as they float by like bubbles. Observe your thoughts with detached interest rather than getting emotionally involved. In your mind, repeat the phrase: "I am not my thoughts." Let the thoughts come and go without holding on. Thoughts themselves can be emotionally charged, but *you* don't have to be when you recognize that you are separate from your thoughts.

Thoughtfulness: WHAT DO YOUR THOUGHTS DO AT NIGHT?

For a lucky few, evening thoughts quiet down and float gently into pleasant dreams, but many of us wake up in the middle of the night with thoughts racing and can't get back to sleep. Tonight, if anxious thoughts awaken you, practice observing your thoughts rather than getting caught up in them. Watch your thoughts pass as if they have nothing to do with you. Notice how they seem more urgent than they do during the day; know that is just an illusion. See the urgent thoughts flowing past you, then imagine that stream of thoughts turning into an actual stream—a gentle bubbling stream winding through a meadow full of flowers warmed by the sun. Trees along the banks rustle in a soft wind. All is as it should be in that moment. Let the sound of that stream lull you back to sleep.

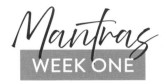

Mantras
WEEK ONE

I notice, without judgment, how I talk to myself, and I gently remind myself that I can be my own loving and compassionate advocate.

———————————

I use my intuition to determine what is healthy for my body, my mind, and my spirit, because nobody knows me better than I know myself.

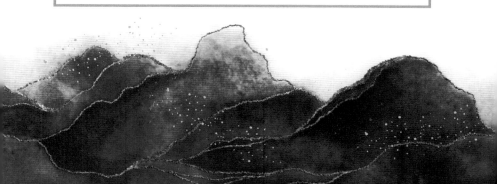

Strengthen Your Closest Relationships

Love is the white light of emotion.

DIANE ACKERMAN

Voice: DO YOUR WORDS LIFT PEOPLE UP OR TEAR THEM DOWN?

How you use your voice can have a greater impact on others than you might realize. What you say can lift someone up or fill someone with self-doubt. Speaking affirming words to the people you love the most is an uplifting gift, but it's easy to make unintentionally disparaging or harsh comments to the people with whom we share our daily lives. How about a positive voice challenge for today? See if you can go for an entire day without saying anything negative, critical, or sarcastic to the person or people you talk with frequently. No "I was just joking" or "I'm just trying to help" or "I'm just pointing out what you could do differently." Today, let your language consist of positive, supportive words only. This exercise can help you become more mindful of how you speak to people, especially those closest to you. Think of this as an opportunity to curate your words so they become more precious and valuable to the people you love.

Voice: HOW POWERFUL ARE YOUR POSITIVE WORDS?

As you wind down for the evening, think about how easy, or how difficult, it was to speak positively to others. Did you find that it took more effort to filter your words to the people with whom you share the closest bond? For some, this is surprisingly challenging. It's easy to take those nearest to us for granted, and when we do so we can become less aware of how our words might impact them. Reflect upon how today's practice felt for you and whether or not it changed the energy between you and the people with whom you interacted in a positive way. Did affirming words given result in affirming words received? Did anyone notice anything different? Think about how sustainable such a habit might be if you practiced it regularly, and what kind of benefits it might reap in your close relationships.

Intuition: THE LOVE
LANGUAGE OF PHYSICAL TOUCH

Humans are exquisitely sensitive to touch, and this responsiveness is a sort of intuition. This is what people mean when they talk about "chemistry" between two people. It's especially important in intimate romantic relationships. Chemistry isn't the only necessary factor in a rewarding intimate relationship. You can have chemistry and the person still may not be right for you for other reasons, but without chemistry, you may find that true intimacy won't be achievable. Chemistry can be applied to platonic relationships as well. There is an inner knowing about why physical contact with some people is so pleasurable and comfortable, while contact with other people isn't, and may feel unpleasant, even if the other person seems perfectly nice. Pay attention to the feelings that come up in response to touch. Even a handshake, a hug, or a peck on the cheek can be triggers for the intuition. You may want to simply ask yourself: Does this person make me feel at ease, or do they alert my self-protective instincts?

Intuition: LISTEN TO WHAT ISN'T BEING SAID

It's nice to spend your evening with someone you love, whether it's a romantic partner or a close family member or friend. When we retreat from the noise of the day and return to the quiet comforts of home, these intimate evening hours can be peaceful times of verbal and physical communion, but they can also be a chance for you to use your intuition to better understand the people closest to you. When the day's distractions are set aside, and it's just you and the person or people you love, try to feel the energy in the room and notice body language and expressions. Is there something more going on than is being said? Do you get a sense that someone you love may be troubled by something but not sharing it? Feeling stronger emotions than they are letting on? Can you pick up on subtle cues that they are pulling away from you, or trying to get closer because they need reassurance? So much communication within intimate relationships is unspoken. Use your intuition to learn even more about your partner and loved ones than you could ever learn from the words they speak out loud.

Balance:

WHO HELPS YOU?

We live in an era that greatly values independence and individual autonomy. I know so many women who are extremely independent: powerful, intelligent, fierce, and capable. And that is amazing! But there is one thing that can be hard to master, or reconcile, when you come into your own power. You may spend all day using your independent energy to run a company or household, manage a team, or take care of others, but do you allow yourself to be helped? For some people, asking for help or feeling that they need someone else can feel like weakness or concession, but the ability to be a little bit vulnerable and admit you can't do it all is actually a strength. In balanced relationships, especially intimate relationships, two people each exercising their skills and strengths in complementary ways can rely on each other as they create endlessly exciting and rewarding experiences together. If you are keeping that from happening because you "have to be strong," I totally get that, and quite possibly, you *could* "do it all." But when you find people you can really trust, letting them gift you with their talents and strengths can be infinitely more satisfying than going it alone.

Balance:

TEST THE WATERS OF VULNERABILITY

Tonight, spend some time contemplating the concept of *vulnerability*. That's a word that scares a lot of people, and being vulnerable *is* scary, especially when it's not your choice. But being purposefully vulnerable is different. It is a willingness to lower your defenses for someone you love and trust. It's certainly not easy, especially if you tend to keep your guard up most of the time and enjoy being independent and autonomous. Yet there is nothing more rewarding in an intimate relationship than opening up the gates of your heart and letting someone else in who has earned your faith and proved they are willing and able to accept, protect, and love all that you are. It's okay to be strong, to be cautious, even to be guarded out there in the wide world. But there will be a small handful of people in life with whom you can share the soft parts of your heart. When you think one of those people has come along, test the waters with moments of willing vulnerability, and see how it can enrich and grow your most intimate relationships.

Rejuvenation: THE POWER OF CLOSE CONNECTION

One of the most surprising things I've learned about rejuvenation in my many years of study and practice is that, while it's true that rejuvenating the body has much to do with lifestyle, rejuvenating the spirit is largely about human connection. Isolation is stressful and can contribute to or worsen illness. Feeling connected, supported, and deeply loved bolsters health and healing as well as mental well-being and feelings of contentment and happiness. It's easy to take our closest and most intimate relationships for granted, but today, see if you can reach out and connect with someone important to you in a more meaningful way. Look them in the eye when they are talking. Make a phone call or, in the case of a romantic partner, send them a playful or sexy text, just to let them know you're thinking of them. Touch them affectionately to show support and attraction. When they speak, turn toward them to actively listen. Feel the warmth and joy that come from spending time with someone who really gets you and wants only the very best for you. There are mental health benefits to being supportive and giving love as well as receiving it. Connection goes both ways, and the power of connection is truly awesome.

Rejuvenation: REFRESHING YOUR ROMANTIC LIFE

Could your sex life use a refresh? Sex itself can be incredibly rejuvenating for relationships, for self-esteem, and for the physical body as it releases pleasure hormones like oxytocin, serotonin, and dopamine. Over the years, couples can get out of the habit of intimate physical contact, especially in long-term relationships, but it's never too late to tap into that rejuvenating power . . . even if you need to schedule it. (Don't let anyone tell you that's not romantic—sometimes it's the only way to make it happen!) Our material belongings require upkeep, our physical bodies thrive when we fuel them with a nourishing diet and exercise, and our sexual and intimate relationships need maintenance and upkeep too. This evening, create an experience that will make someone you love feel truly seen and cared for. Go out to a nice dinner (your treat?), cook a romantic meal at home, or order in from your favorite spot. Talk and listen. Really focus on each other without distractions. Whether you go all out or you just bask in the reassuring contact of cuddling, intimate interaction with a trusted and caring partner can make you feel more confident, more energetic, and glow-ier.

Abundance: YOU'RE ALREADY RICH IN LOVE

For people who aren't currently in a supportive and rewarding romantic relationship, it can feel like everyone else has love. But there are different kinds of love, all of which create a foundation for intimate relationships and can be just as rewarding as the closeness found in romance. Remember that love also lives within *you*. Cultivate your inner love abundance by practicing loving yourself, getting really clear on what you want in a relationship, and working on becoming someone who doesn't *need* a relationship but who is fully formed and content from within. How can someone who is a good match for you find you and recognize you as the perfect match for them if you don't know and love yourself? Start by acknowledging the truth that you are worthy of love, then feel the love abundance growing inside of you until it spills out of you like a beacon. When you enrich the love you offer yourself, you enrich the love you're able to give to others. If you are already in a relationship, this will also enrich and improve the quality of the love you have to give.

Abundance : CONTEMPLATE
THE LOVE IN YOUR LIFE

This evening, spend some time sitting with the concept of *love abundance*. What does that mean to you? What is your definition of love? If you don't currently have a fulfilling intimate or romantic relationship in your life, do you feel an emotional deficit from this, or do you still feel love-abundant? If you are in a healthy and satisfying romantic relationship, are you giving all the love you can to that person, and are you receiving enough in return to feel deeply supported and cherished? Love comes in many forms, and cultivating a mentality around love *abundance* rather than love *scarcity* can help you better receive and offer affection. Let your mind wander as you think about love and get a sense of where you sit with the idea. As you drift off to sleep, repeat the words: *Love is abundant. It flows from me and flows to me, and its source is infinite.*

Nurturing:
ALLOW OTHERS TO CARE FOR YOU

Nurturing is a two-way street. When you nurture some-one, you will often find that they have the impulse to nurture you back. If you've ever been comforted or soothed by a child, someone for whom you are a caregiver, or even an animal, you can see firsthand that the nurturing behavior you are model-ing is having a positive effect. You may be a natural nurturer, but if you resist receiving nurturing from others, consider why. Perhaps your instinct is to give rather than to receive, or perhaps allowing others to care for you makes you feel too vulnerable, which can be daunting. However, when you accept nurturing without resistance or immediate reciprocation, you allow other people to grow in their own ability to nurture others. Think of how good you feel when you are able to nurture someone. Letting someone take care of you is giving them the gift of that same positive feeling. Moreover, by learning to accept being nurtured as well as nurturing, you will be making the world a more nurturing place for all.

Nurturing:
OFFER UNCONDITIONAL LOVE

It's easy to think you know how someone else should behave, to point out mistakes, judge, or try to change someone. But if you really want to make a person feel safe and loved, accepting them for exactly who they are—*right now*—is the way to do it. It's important to note that who someone *is* isn't the same as what they *do*. Think about how accepting you are of the faults you perceive in those you love the most. There will always be tension between you and someone whom you think should be different than they are. You don't have to approve of, or even tolerate, destructive or harmful behavior, but when you fully accept someone—a child, a parent, a friend, and especially your primary partner—that's powerful. Ironically, thinking someone should become better in your eyes can make it harder for them to become better in their own eyes. Accepting them and fully supporting *their* efforts to grow, rather than your efforts to change them, can help them feel the confidence and nurturing support they need to make the choices that will create the outcomes they desire. Showing someone that your love is unconditional is one of the greatest gifts you can give.

Thoughtfulness:
TAKE A BREAK FROM TECHNOLOGY

How often do you interact with your loved ones without technology? Couples and families often get into a rut on the weekends: distracted meals, all-day media consumption, text conversations, and barely any eye contact or physical touch. Today, try taking the day off from media. It's Sunday, so do you really need to check those work messages? Do you actually want to turn on the television, or is it just a habit? How might you and your loved ones spend the day together, free from screens and electronics? You could take a day trip, a nature hike, have a picnic, ride bicycles, read together, or take a long leisurely walk holding hands. You could cook a special dinner together or go out to a new restaurant you haven't tried. (Can you find one that isn't plastered with televisions?) Or you could just spend a quiet day together, talking, cuddling, and reconnecting. This can be incredibly rejuvenating for your relationships and give your brain a much-needed break from the technology you will surely need to reengage with tomorrow.

Thoughtfulness: GET CURIOUS ABOUT SOMEONE YOU KNOW WELL

Tonight, spend some time intentionally thinking about your partner or another person you're close to. Who are they, totally separate from who they are *to you* and who they are *for you*? Who are they, in and of themselves? Have you ever really considered that question? What are their unique personality traits or gifts? How do you think they see themselves? There is always something new to learn about people, even if you know them very well. Take some time to wonder about their dreams, their disappointments, what might have happened in their past. What drives them? What moves them? What makes them angry or joyful or sad? Curiosity is at the heart of compelling conversations. Ask them questions about themselves and really listen to their answers, for a deeper emotional connection. We are infinitely complex creatures, and no matter how well you know someone, there is always more to learn. Let this exercise in thoughtfulness increase your intimacy.

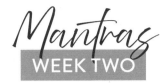

Mantras
WEEK TWO

I open my heart to an abundance of love, friendship, and connection.

I nurture the people I love by giving them my undistracted time and attention.

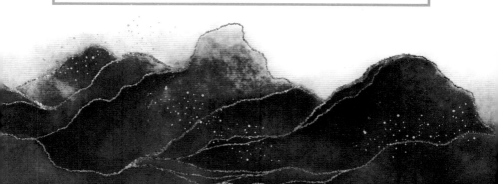

Get Connected with Your Community

True self-respect, being very different from false pride, leads inevitably to respecting others.

VIRGINIA MOORE

Voice: TURN YOUR INNER VOICE OUTWARD

During Week One, we explored your inner voice and examined how you talk to yourself. Your inner voice is influenced by whether you are alone or with other people. When you're isolated, it makes sense that your focus, and your inner voice, go inward, centering on how *you* feel. But too much self-focus can become unhealthy, even oppressive or paralyzing, over time. We all need some alone time for relaxation and self-reflection, but when we connect to others, we can balance that inner *I* with an inner *you* in ways that can result in actions that reach out and allow us to be of service to others. "What do *you* need from me?" "How can I help *you*?" "I'm here to listen to *you*." And in a beautiful twist, that "you" focus can be just what your inner "I" really needs.

Voice: CREATE
OPPORTUNITIES TO LISTEN

The counterpart to talking is listening. How well did you do this today? Think back over those hours, to all the times when you were listening rather than talking. What did you learn about your family members, coworkers, neighbors, and friends, just by hearing the words swirling around you? If you realize that you didn't listen very well, think about how you might practice this skill tomorrow. Use your voice to prompt opportunities for listening, without any plan for offering your point of view or as an excuse to tell your own stories. You can do this by asking open-ended questions like: "How are things going for you lately?" "What's new in your life?" "What are you spending your time on these days?" "Is there anything that you could use some help with?" Once you ask, really listen to what that person says, without judgment or interruption. Resist the urge to take your turn talking about yourself, or to try to fix the other person's problems. You don't have to offer a solution, and the person talking might not even want one. Just be there, with open ears and an open heart.

Intuition:
GOOD CONNECTIONS

As people grow, change, and move through different stages of life, some friends may be there all along. Others may come into your life at certain times and then fall away as your paths diverge. But we don't always choose our friends consciously, and we might hang on to certain people out of habit, rather than intention. We may keep people in our lives even though we no longer get along with them very well, or when the connection begins to feel more exhausting than joyful and fulfilling. If this sounds familiar, it might be time to do a "friend audit." Make a list of all the people you currently consider to be your friends, then carefully scan the list and listen to your intuition. When you see the name of someone and it fills you with a warm, happy feeling, that's a keeper. If a name gives you a sense of discomfort, anger, annoyance, or dread, even if you can't express exactly why, it may be time to politely back off from that friendship. It's probably not serving your highest good, or the other person's.

Intuition: WHO MAKES YOU A BETTER VERSION OF YOURSELF?

As you wind down for the evening, keep thinking about all the people in your life. Some you know well, others you may know only casually, but no matter how close the relationship, your intuition knows more than your conscious awareness. Deep within, you are an excellent judge of character, so as you think about the people in your life, including those you hope to stay connected with forever and those who may just be here for a season, let your intuition be your guide. Who makes your life richer? Who inspires you to set better goals? Who tempts you into behaviors that don't serve you or others well? Who makes you feel down or brings out your worst side? There are reasons for all of these effects other people have on you. Even if you don't know them consciously, your intuition knows. If you aren't sure about someone, sit quietly for a few minutes and ponder whether they help you become a better version of yourself. Let your intuition speak to you, and trust what you hear.

Balance: PERSONALLY CAPABLE AND COMMUNALLY CONNECTED

Humans are built to be both autonomous and interdependent. To feel balanced, we need to be both personally capable and communally connected. You may have heard that self-worth should come from within, but nobody exists in a bubble. The truth is that your sense of self-worth is healthiest when it comes from a balanced perspective. If you depend entirely on others for your self-worth, you give away your power. If you rely only on yourself, you may block that valuable connectedness and awareness of how impactful on your own sense of self it is to be useful and of service to others. You should know that you have inherent dignity and are worthy of love, but don't forget that we all rely on one another, and reaching out to see what others need is one of the best ways to boost your own morale.

Balance : CONNECTION
WITH OTHERS ISN'T ALWAYS EASY

As you look back over your day, see if you can pinpoint moments of connection with others. Were there high and low points, triumphs and mistakes, connections and fractures? These are all natural parts of the emotional wave that characterizes relationships with other human beings. Everyone is different and complex, and relationships won't always be characterized by harmony, but connection is vital for a sense of fulfillment and happiness. Especially with those who seem very different from you, finding ways to communicate peacefully and charitably can be particularly rewarding when you realize that, no matter how distinct you may seem and how disparate your opinions may be, there is a golden thread that connects us all—one that shimmers when we treat the bonds between ourselves and others with honor and respect.

Rejuvenation: CREATE A LIFE OUTSIDE OF YOUR HOME

In this modern era of isolation due to ubiquitous digital access and an endless landscape of distraction, it can become all too easy to focus on yourself and your immediate family and forget that you are part of a community. But isolation isn't good for mental health. Humans have spent most of their time on this earth relying on one another for survival, and close-knit groups, clans, tribes, and eventually communities were the center of life. This is why it's wearing on the human psyche to be isolated. We simply didn't evolve that way. But knowing this means you can choose to enjoy the rejuvenating effects of participating in community. Discover ways to get involved with local groups or causes that you support. The mental stimulation and social enjoyment you can get from connecting to people outside of your own household can deepen and enrich the life that takes place within the walls of your home as well.

Rejuvenation: HOW WELL DO YOU SERVE YOUR COMMUNITY?

This evening, spend some time reflecting on yourself as part of a community. Who are you to others? Who are you to your friends, colleagues, and neighbors? Imagine seeing yourself from the point of view of others who don't live with you. Look nonjudgmentally, as a compassionate observer. Is there anything you'd like to work on, considering your role in people's lives from a broader perspective? Are there ways you might strengthen some of your less well-tended social connections, or things you could do to be a better friend or community member? Does this exercise help you to discover or define any potential new interests or priorities? To see yourself as a part of a bigger network of people can change your perspective in a rejuvenating way.

Abundance: TURN
LONELINESS INTO NEW CONNECTIONS

Making friends might have seemed easy in your twenties, but many of those bonds can weaken, or disintegrate entirely, as people start families and their emphasis shifts away from friends in favor of deepening love and family relationships. Later in life—when children grow up and move out, a romantic partner is no longer with you, or your friends have moved on to different stages of their own lives—you may find yourself feeling lonely. Change is difficult and loneliness is common, even if you have people around you, especially if your relationships don't feel deep or meaningful. Perhaps this season is an opportunity for you to focus once again on building abundant friendships. Try reconnecting with old friends to catch up and create new opportunities to get together. Reach out to potential new friends if you feel a connection. If initiating contact feels intimidating, a good first step is to find an opportunity to do things with like-minded people, like joining a group focused on an activity you enjoy. These new or revived connections can do wonders to restore you with an abundant feeling of emotional richness.

Abundance:
SHARE YOUR GIFTS

Something about the act of giving turns the attention outward in a way that can take the mind off problems and too much self-reflection. While it's true many people give until they are drained and really do need to focus on self-care, giving doesn't have to be, and indeed should not be, depleting. It should fill you up and energize you. The secret is to give where you are most abundant, rather than trying to pull from where you have the least energy. What are your greatest resources? If you have too much time, try giving some of it away by volunteering. If you are brimming with creativity, can you offer your gifts to a group who needs someone who can write, draw, or do graphic design? If you have financial resources, where might you donate that can do the most good to serve a cause you believe in? If you are a natural caretaker, could you spend some time visiting the elderly, reading to children, or taking care of animals? Whatever it is you love to do, focus your giving there, and feel the power of sharing your abundant gifts.

Nurturing: DIFFERENT
PEOPLE HAVE DIFFERENT NEEDS

An important and often-overlooked aspect of nurturing is *not* to treat others as you would like to be treated, but instead, to treat others the way *they* would like to be treated. This may not be the golden rule, but it is a more intentionally loving way to relate to others because it shows you notice and consider who they are as a unique individual and not just as a reflection of yourself. What makes your partner, your child, or your friend feel safest and most loved? Their needs may not be the same as yours. If you aren't sure, just ask. The question itself is a way to nurture, but the follow-through is the most important part. Gift someone with the kind of support and care they most need and desire.

Nurturing: WHEN NURTURING MEANS *NOT* DOING SOMETHING

It's natural—and admirable—to feel called to action when someone is in need of support, but sometimes what that person most requires is for us to hold back words, actions, and judgments. This evening, think about how your words and efforts affect others by seeing yourself being the recipient of those words or actions. If you realize that you may sometimes speak or act without this awareness, try applying the thoughtfulness litmus test. Before saying anything, ask yourself: "Might this hurt someone?" If the answer is probably, maybe, or even if you aren't sure, then consider not saying it or offering only kindness instead. See if this changes the dynamic in your relationships.

Thoughtfulness:
SMALL GESTURES OF SELF-SACRIFICE

One especially meaningful way to be more thoughtful is to do something that someone else wants you to do, even when you don't really feel like it. While it's important to make sure you're investing time and energy into your self-care, putting someone else's needs ahead of your own (only when it doesn't harm you or deplete you) can be a beautiful expression of your love for them. Even the seemingly smallest gestures can have deeply felt impacts on our relationships. Attending a stuffy work event with your sweetheart? Staying up late to bake cookies for the school bake sale? Listening to your child's very, very long story without looking at your phone? Supporting a friend's ambitions, rather than criticizing their outrageous idea? It may feel like you always put everyone else first, and that's probably true, but where can you make a gesture today that only costs you a little but would mean the world to another person?

Thoughtfulness: CAST YOUR NET OF KINDNESS EVEN WIDER

How broadly do you cast your net of thoughtfulness? Most people at least try to behave thoughtfully towards the people that matter to them, and surely you show compassion and support to those you love. But just imagine how different a place the world would be if we all extended just a fraction of that same thoughtfulness to people we don't know, or even to people we don't necessarily like. As you lie down to rest this evening, think about some ways you can intentionally make offerings of kindness to strangers throughout the day tomorrow. Open the door for someone at a coffee shop, let another car ahead of you in traffic, offer a friendly greeting and a kind word to someone who looks a little down. Over time, these small, intentional gestures of kindness become a habitual way of being that can bless others with a sense that people really are kind after all. They can make *you* feel surprisingly good, too.

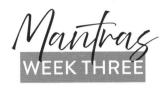

WEEK THREE

I give support and encouragement
to all those around me, and I
willingly receive it in return.

_____

I am more than myself. I am more
than my family. I am a member of
the human race, and there is more
to connect us than to divide us.

Recapture the Whimsy of Childhood

What one loves in childhood stays in the heart forever.

MARY JO PUTNEY

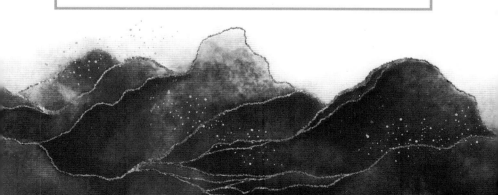

Voice:

GREET YOUR CHILD SELF

When you were a child, you saw the world with fresh eyes. As an adult, you see the world through the lens of wisdom gained from experience. But what if you could meet *yourself* as a child? What would you say to that child with so much life ahead of them? If you can, find a childhood photo of yourself, or think about what you looked like at a young age. Sit quietly, close your eyes, and imagine taking that child's hand and sitting together. What do you want to tell that little boy or girl? What lessons, encouragements, or warnings might you impart? Express the love and compassion you have for that little child, and for the adult they'll grow up to be.

Voice:

LET YOUR INNER CHILD SPEAK

Today, you meditated on what you would say to yourself as a child. This evening, complete that conversation. Sit quietly, close your eyes, and imagine meeting that child again. This time, ask your child self what they want to say to *you*, as you are now. What wide-eyed wisdom does your younger self have that might remind you of your purpose and potential? What are that child's fears, hopes, and dreams for you? Imagine how this conversation would go, as you let your younger self speak to you. Are there things you still believe or that you're still passionate about? Are there things you've forgotten or lost that you might revisit as an adult? Let your inner child speak and see what you can learn.

Intuition:

A CHILD'S SENSE OF KNOWING

Children have an amazing intuitive sense that can be dulled along the path to and through adulthood, yet somewhere deep down that childlike intuition remains. Today, see if you can tap into the sense of knowing that once came so easily to you. Remember what the world felt like when you were a child, and see if you can access that point of view again. How did you think about yourself? How did you see other people? How did you feel about the place you lived? What were your most beloved things to do? Was the world a more magical place back then? Did you see and experience things differently before you felt the need to manage or try to control the circumstances that created your reality? See if you can look back through those eyes. How does your life look different right now, when you view it from a more childlike perspective? What does your intuition tell you about what you need, or what you need to change?

Intuition:
SPEND A MOMENT IN YOUR MEMORY

This evening, without expectation or judgment, close your eyes and spend some time imagining yourself as a child again. Choose an age you remember at least fairly well, or an event that you recall experiencing before you went through puberty. Just remember. What details can you identify about your surroundings, the other people present, and your sense of self? What did your reality feel like? What did it feel like before you had to earn a living, before you had your own family, adult friends, and adult life filled with responsibilities? Let yourself live inside this memory for a while and see what comes up intuitively for you. Try to identify at least one feeling related to this experience that you would like to recapture. Is there anything you feel you've lost, a point of view you forgot you used to have, or a feeling you could re-experience?

Balance:

EQUILIBRIUM IS ACTIVE

When people think of balance, they often imagine a static state of perfect harmony, where all the disparate parts of life exist in a harmonious equilibrium. But that's not what balance is really like. When you were a child, did you ever ride on a teeter-totter at the playground? (Maybe you called it a seesaw.) The goal of a fun time on a teeter-totter isn't to get both people to balance in perfect stillness with their feet off the ground. The goal is to go up and down: with every up, the other side goes down, and with every down, the other side goes up. Think of this as a metaphor for your life. When you are up, you know you'll be going down next, and when you are down, you know you're about to head up. That's what real balance looks like. It's active, not static, and it's always changing.

Balance:

HOW DO YOU WIND DOWN?

What was your nighttime routine as a child? Try to recall the details. How was it different than your bedtime routine today? What time did you go to bed? Did you have a favorite pair of pajamas? Do you remember what kind of bedding you had? Did you always, or never, wear slippers? Did you have a bedtime snack? A fanciful toothbrush or a certain brand of toothpaste? Did you settle down with a bedtime story? What was your bed like? Did you share your room with a sibling and whisper together after the lights were out, or did you have your own room and a special toy to cuddle? Did you read a book beneath a lamp's yellow glow or under the covers with a flashlight? What can you do to recapture some of that childhood wonder? An earlier bedtime perhaps, or your old bedtime snack? How about actually wearing pajamas, or reading a bedtime story, or even finding something to cuddle with? Balancing your adult bedtime routine with the one you used to have as a child can make going to bed feel more appealing and might result in a more pleasant routine that feels less burdened by the pressures of adulthood.

Rejuvenation:
A BEGINNER'S MIND

The world is filled with interesting things, fascinating people, spectacular places, and opportunities for pure wonder, but if you aren't seeing the world with fresh eyes, try adopting a beginner's mind. This is a concept borrowed from Zen Buddhism that means experiencing something with a clear, open mind and no preconceptions, as if you—like a child—were an absolute beginner. Learning things about the world with a beginner's mind can rejuvenate your passion for life and your excitement about new things. Look to the day ahead. Can you move through it with a beginner's mind? Try to notice that first morning sip of aromatic tea or rich coffee, the sounds of nature outside your window, the music you listen to when you exercise or commute to work. While you do your work, interact with people, eat your meals, drive your car, or whatever else you do on a typical day, can you come into the present moment and see it with fresh eyes? Could this new perspective inspire your curiosity or creativity? Let your mind expand into the possibilities of all the things you haven't yet learned about the world, about life, and even about yourself.

Rejuvenation: BREATHE
NEW LIFE INTO THE ORDINARY

How did you do today, trying to see the world with a beginner's mind? Look back over the day and consider when you were on automatic pilot and when you were able to step out of your routine and into a more mindful state. This takes practice, so even if you didn't do it very often today, think about how you might continue this practice tomorrow. Did you focus on finding opportunities to stop and really savor the present moment as if for the first time? See if you can continue to have a beginner's mind this evening. Focus on what you notice as you wind down your day. The soothing relief of removing your shoes when you return home in the evening. The way the world looks outside as the sun sets. The smell and taste of dinner. The interactions with family or friends. Your typical day is a collection of so many unique moments. How can you mindfully experience each one to see it with fresh eyes? This can be a lifelong practice that never gets old because it's always about seeing things anew.

Abundance:

HOW DO YOU SPEND YOUR FREE TIME?

Once we hit the ground running as adults, the idea of free time can seem like a luxury of childhood. And yet, "free time," or time during which you have nothing you *have* to do, is a valuable resource. How do you spend yours? Even if you only get a limited amount of free time, approaching it with an abundance mindset can help you make the most of every moment. If you waste it on mindless activities that don't relax you and that you barely remember (social media scrolling? bad television?), you can't reap the significant benefits of free time spent in ways that enrich your life. How you spend your spare time should fill you up in ways that are edifying and equip you with the physical, emotional, and mental energy you need to be fully present in your daily life. Spend some time thinking about how you will spend your free time today, especially if you don't get many of those precious moments.

Abundance:

YOUR FIRST FRIENDS

Just as we find ourselves with less free time in adulthood, we may also come to realize that the circle of friends we consider real and true has shrunken to a smaller, but still cherished, group. Tonight, devote a bit of time to remembering the friends who populated your childhood. As the old song goes, "Make new friends, but keep the old. One is silver and the other gold." Meditate on one of your first friends in childhood who taught you something or changed you in some positive way. Picture this person the way you remember them. Think about how they looked, talked, and moved. What brought you together? What are some of the experiences you shared? How did they help shape the person you grew up to be? Childhood friendships often contain clues for the kinds of connections we value most. Did that early friendship establish standards or patterns you still look for in new friends? Spending time thinking about an early friendship can help you shed light on your friendships now and reflect on your friendship abundance, which is rooted in quality over quantity.

Nurturing: WHO IS YOUR CARETAKING ROLE MODEL?

Your nurturing style has likely been influenced by the kind of nurturing you received as a child. Some people are natural nurturers, and others have a harder time tapping into this skill set. If you struggle in this area, it can be useful to look back at the kind of care you received as a child, which likely influenced how you learned to nurture others. If the people who reared you weren't comfortable with nurturing, you may not be either, but rest assured that you can *nurture* your nurturing skills. The key is simply to show interest in and encourage someone's growth and goals. There are many role models out there. Think of someone whose nurturing style you admire; maybe they've supported your own growth and goals, or maybe you've just observed how they care for others. Think about specific things they do, encouraging words they say, how they express themselves, and then . . . practice! It may feel awkward at first, but the more you do it, the more natural it will feel.

Nurturing: THE PROFOUND POWER OF A BATH

Few things are more nurturing than a bath, and—in a most beautiful way—our relationship with this ritual changes with the circle of life. When you were a baby, your parent or guardian lovingly bathed you with gentle attention, and eventually taught you to care for yourself in this same way. If you become a parent, you do the same for your children. Eventually, the people who once bathed you may grow to an age where they require your assistance in return. As will you, one day. Something about the feel of the warm water, the vulnerable act of cleansing, and the physical touch is profound in its ability to calm, reassure, and rinse away stress. Even washing someone's hair or feet can be an act of pure love. This evening, whether for yourself or for a loved one who needs assistance, pay extra attention to the loving and nurturing process of caring for the physical body in this gentle way. Along with the day's dirt and germs, imagine that you are also washing away stress, anxiety, and worry as you honor the body that you've been given and create a clean slate for another day.

Thoughtfulness:
THE STORY OF YOUR CHILDHOOD

The stories we read as children become a part of us in a lasting and powerful way. Can you recall some of your favorite books from childhood? What about them made such an impact on your young mind and heart? A sense of adventure or imagination? A feeling of wistfulness or maybe a little mischief? If you were going to write a book about yourself as a child, how would you describe the main character? What do they want? What's standing in their way, and how will they overcome these obstacles to get it? Actually writing down stories of your life can be an illuminating practice. Just thinking about the way you used to view the world may trigger memories and discoveries about why you are who you are today. Don't worry about how well you write. Nobody has to see it. Tell the stories with as much detail as you can remember. The point is the process, not the result. This exercise is just for you, to help you reflect on the events that have shaped you. (Although, who knows . . . this could be the start of your memoir!)

Thoughtfulness:
DREAMS AND NIGHTMARES

I like to think of dreams as stories that our brains tell us while we sleep. Do you remember any dreams you had as a child? Children have some of the most vivid and memorable (and sometimes scary) dreams that may stick with them for life. This evening, think about the dreams you remember from childhood, and thoughtfully apply your adult wisdom to interpreting them. What emotion was present in the dreams? Do you recall what you were going through at the time that might have led to those particular visions? Do you still have any dreams that are similar or recurring? Based on the dreams you remember, see if you can come up with some insights into who you were then and who you are today.

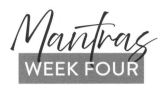

Mantras
WEEK FOUR

My inner child is precious, and I cherish, nurture, love, and protect that child from harm.

———————————

I view the world with a sense of wonder and a beginner's mind.

Let Your Body Tell You What It Needs

Life itself is the proper binge.

JULIA CHILD

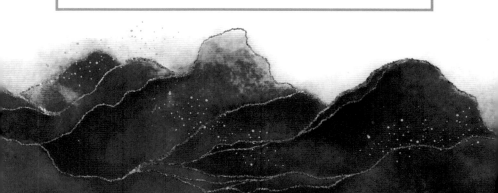

Voice:

YOUR BODY'S LANGUAGE

Your body has a voice, and it is speaking to you all the time. Every ache, pain, twinge, twitch, and cramp. All of your digestive sensations and hunger pangs. Each slight mood dip and overwhelmingly good feeling. That surge of energy and sudden wave of fatigue. Every sneeze, every cough, every laugh, every sob. These are all messages from your inside to your outside. Your body speaks a language just for you, and it can inform you of much that you may not consciously recognize at first, including when you are truly hungry and when you are emotionally hungry, when you need to move your body and when you need to rest, and so much more about your physical and mental health. Today, be aware of all the physical and emotional sensations you experience, and what your body might be trying to tell you about how to keep yourself healthy, nourished, and strong.

Voice: WHAT DID YOUR BODY TELL YOU TODAY?

Look back over your day and think about the physical sensations you noticed. Did your body let you know in subtle ways that certain things you were eating were good for you or bad for you? Did it tell you when you were overdoing exercise, or were there physical discomforts related to too much sitting? Did you feel urges to eat or to stop eating, to move or to be still? What made you feel good? What made you feel bad? When you are tuned in to your body, you don't need a diet or exercise plan—your body already has one for you. You only need to pay attention in order to follow it. The more you notice and heed those signals, the more you will learn what is truly the healthiest way for you, personally, to live—a way that may not apply to anyone else, but that is specially designed just for *you*.

Intuition:

WHAT IS INTUITIVE EATING?

Intuitive eating is a way of consuming food and drinks based on intuition rather than externally imposed diet rules. This is an enjoyable and natural way to eat that doesn't restrict but instead helps you learn to follow your intuition about what and how much you really want to take in. Today, continue the practice of listening to your body that we began yesterday, and use it to try eating intuitively. Pay attention to your hunger and cues of satiety. If you aren't hungry, don't eat. If you are hungry, think about what your body actually craves, then eat it slowly, deliberately, and mindfully, enjoying every bite, until you feel that you've had enough. Notice what foods you truly enjoy and what you eat just because you think you should. When you tell yourself you can always eat if you want to and you can have any food you desire, you may realize that the allure of "forbidden" foods fades away. This style of eating has helped many people conquer compulsive eating and overeating tendencies because restriction and deprivation are often what cause these problems in the first place. It can take some practice, but once you learn to eat intuitively, it feels great and you may discover your appetite and weight regulate themselves effortlessly.

Intuition: HOW DOES YOUR BODY WANT TO MOVE?

Intuitive movement is similar to intuitive eating, in that you don't follow a prescribed exercise plan but instead follow your intuition about when you really need to move and when you should rest. Do whatever movement feels natural and is enjoyable—walking, cycling, yoga, dance, stretching, weight-lifting, or even just running around all day getting things done and having fun. With intuitive movement, you learn to feel and honor your body's requests. This is how humans have lived for thousands of years. Now that life is less physically strenuous, we may need to find more opportunities for movement that makes us feel strong and healthy, but exercise should feel natural, not punishing. Think about how you might move more intuitively tomorrow, whether that's taking some time out for an exercise you enjoy or just finding ways to be more active and mobile throughout the day.

Balance:

LET'S TAKE IT LITERALLY

Balance is an often-overlooked but important aspect of functional movement because it helps to keep us safe. To maintain a sense of balance and avoid falls and fractures, it should be something everyone practices throughout life. One good way to hone and maintain balance is with yoga poses that require standing on one foot—such as the tree pose, in which you stand on one foot and place the sole of your other foot on the inside thigh of your standing leg. But you don't need to do yoga to practice balance. Today, whenever you think of it, stand on one foot and see how long you can balance, then switch feet and try again. If you feel unsteady, practice next to a wall or something you can hold on to if necessary. Do this periodically throughout the day—and every day—and you will strengthen the muscles in your feet, ankles, and legs, which could someday prevent a serious injury.

Balance:

THE VIBRANT TRIAD

The Vibrant Triad is a system I use to help people achieve balance in the three foundational areas that largely determine health and wellness: what you eat, how you move, and how you connect with others. Miss any of these three foundations and your triangle will be incomplete. Within the triangle, there are other triangles. A balanced meal or snack will contain some of all three macronutrients: protein, fat, and carbs. Balanced movement includes cardiovascular exercise (like walking, swimming, or biking), strength training (lifting weights, or your own body weight), and stretching (to lengthen and tone muscles and keep joints lubricated). Connection, too, has its own triangle: connection with self, connection with others, and connection with something beyond and greater than yourself, whatever that means to you. Balance your triad, and the triads within each triad, and you can achieve meaningful and vibrant wellness.

Rejuvenation:
EAT YOUR WAY TO GLOWING SKIN

Have you ever considered eating as a way to rejuvenate your skin? There are many ways to rejuvenate skin from the outside, but what you eat can have an even more noticeable effect, from the inside. The best foods for rejuvenating the body contain lubricating healthful fats and antioxidant polyphenols and carotenoids that fight skin-damaging free radicals. My top ten rejuvenating foods are fatty fish (like salmon), avocados, walnuts, eggs, any berries (but especially blueberries and raspberries), broccoli, red bell peppers, sweet potatoes, dark leafy greens (like spinach and kale), and green tea. How many of these foods can you fit into your diet today?

Rejuvenation:
GET TOPSY-TURVY

One fun way to turn back the clock is through inversions. Inversions reverse the effect of gravity on your body, deliver more nutrients to your brain, and bring life and color back into your face. When you are upright all the time, blood can pool in the legs and feet, and inversions help to move it out of your lower extremities. This enhances circulation, gets lymph flowing, relieves bloating and swelling, and even flips your mood upside down. Inversions are also a nice way to wind down at the end of the day. I recommend spending at least five minutes every day in an inversion, for rejuvenation you can feel *and* see. If you are an advanced yoga practitioner, a daily headstand or handstand against the wall will do the trick, but easier poses include lying against a wall, comfortably supported by pillows or bolsters, with your hips scooted forward and your legs up the wall. Or you can lie on the edge of the bed or a bench and hang your head and shoulders off the side. You can also sit upside-down in a chair with your legs over the back of the chair and your head hanging down toward the floor, or just bend over and let your arms and legs hang toward the floor. Find something within your ability that's comfortable and relax there, breathing quietly. Gravity will do the rest.

Abundance:

USE ENERGY TO CREATE ENERGY

Have you ever wondered how your body makes energy? It all comes from microscopic organelles inside your cells called *mitochondria*. These energy factories take the nutrients from the food you eat and turn them into adenosine triphosphate, or ATP, which your body uses as fuel. If you want an abundance of energy, you can send signals to your mitochondria to make more ATP, and even to make more mitochondria. Perhaps counterintuitively, the best way to do this is to *use* energy. Mitochondria are highly responsive to what you do. When you use your muscles, for example, the mitochondria in your muscle cells get the signal that you need energy, so they begin producing more. Sit around all day and your mitochondria get the message that you don't need as much energy, so they produce less. Your muscles contain a lot of mitochondria, and this is precisely why exercise gives people more energy! As long as you give yourself recovery time afterward, movement is the best way to increase your energy abundance. Can you get active today so your mitochondria know to produce more energy for you to use?

Abundance: YOU'RE IN CONTROL OF YOUR CONSUMPTION

Do you feel abundant when you eat? Many people have a scarcity mindset when they eat, meaning that, even if they know logically that there is plenty of food available, something inside them makes them rush through food and eat more than they need or even really want. This mindset can come from instinct (in human history, we may have had to fight to get enough food), as well as from childhood experiences. To help overcome this way of thinking, practice an abundance mindset around food. Before you begin eating, consciously tell yourself: *There is no hurry. There is enough. I can eat slowly and savor this meal. I can stop whenever I want. I can always choose a different food next time. I can always eat more later.* This conscious practice can help you feel more mindful and in control of your food consumption.

Nurturing:
NURTURE WITH NOURISHMENT

Does food equal love? You may or may not have grown up in a household with someone who pushed food on you whether you wanted it or not because that person thought that feeding you was an act of love. While stuffing kids full of sweets and junk food certainly isn't helpful (or healthful), in many ways, food *is* an expression of love because it is the means by which parents nourish their children. The question is: What *kind* of food is the most loving and nurturing for others, as well as for yourself? Food with actual nutritional value, of course. You can nourish the soul *and* the body with foods that come from nature, rather than a factory. Fresh fruits and vegetables, beans and nuts and seeds, fresh fish and pastured meat and eggs—these are all real foods humans are designed to eat. Refined sugar and flour and oil, anything fried or fast—those foods are neither nourishing nor nurturing. So yes, you *can* nurture your loved ones with food. Just remember that to nurture is to nourish.

Nurturing:
WIND DOWN THE DAY

Movement doesn't have to be strenuous. Instead, it can be gentle and nurturing. One of the most self-nurturing activities you can do is the yoga pose called child's pose. To try this pose, kneel on a yoga mat or blanket, feet together, knees apart. Sit back toward your heels and bend forward until you are resting on the ground. Rest your forehead on your folded arms, or on the ground if you extend your arms behind you. Relax into this position, letting your hips sink down between your feet, and allow your torso to rest on the floor. The position should be very comfortable, so if it's not, you can use pillows under your hips, stomach, or head to support yourself. Breathe slowly and deeply and let your stress drain away. This is a comforting pose that is perfect to help you wind down at the end of the day.

Thoughtfulness:
MOVE MORE, THINK BETTER

I've always been fascinated by the research that shows moving while learning things helps people to retain information longer, think more creatively, and understand more easily.[1] Movement generally improves executive brain function in multiple ways, and that is just one of many great reasons to get up and move around during the day. Whether you are listening to a stimulating podcast or audiobook while exercising, or walking with a friend while discussing something you've read, watched, or studied, moving can boost your learning power. Today, when you are working on something you want to remember, try moving around, or at least standing up. Even a brainstorming session on the phone may be more productive if you take a stroll while talking.

Thoughtfulness: WERE YOU GOOD TO YOUR BODY TODAY?

Part of learning how to eat and move intuitively is thoughtful reflection. This evening, take some time to think back over the day. What did you consume and what drove your eating decisions? Think about how much you moved, and how that's reflected in the way your body feels at this very moment. Did you move more or less than your body wanted to? Were your eating and movement decisions based on what your body told you it needed? Or were your choices driven by other things, such as advertising, what other people were doing, self-imposed food rules, or a strenuous schedule that prioritized other responsibilities? The more you become aware of what drives your lifestyle choices, the more you will become conscious of them and able to make decisions more in line with how you want to feel and live.

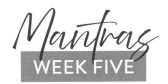

Mantras
WEEK FIVE

I move my body with grace,
gratitude, and self-love.

I eat with reverence, mindfully choosing
the foods that will nourish me, and
considering and experiencing every bite.

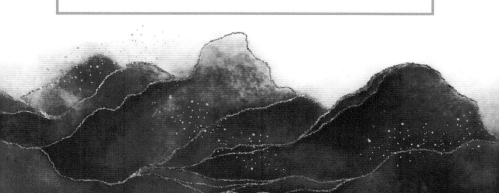

Sleep Well, Dream Big

Happiness consists in getting enough sleep.

ROBERT A. HEINLEIN

Voice:

YOUR MORNING GREETING

What does the voice in your head say to you first thing in the morning? Whatever it is sets the tone for the day. Does that voice say something like, *Oh no, another day of work. I don't want to get out of bed*? Or does that voice look forward to the day ahead with gratitude? This morning, pay attention to that voice in your head that greets you when you awaken. Did you sleep well? Did you eat a healthful meal the evening before? Did you grab your phone and start scrolling before you even got out of bed? All these things can influence how you talk to yourself in the morning, so choose your morning activities wisely. Wait to look at your phone; instead, spend some time stretching, perhaps meditating or praying, setting your intentions for the day, and stepping outside for a moment of fresh air and sunshine, all of which can recalibrate negative self-talk and help you feel more confident and positive about the day to come.

Voice:

THE POWER OF A PRAYER

You could say that prayer is meditation with a voice. Whereas meditation turns your attention inward (even if you speak a mantra), prayer turns your attention outward, as you speak to something greater—whatever higher power or force you connect with. Studies show that both meditation and prayer have similar benefits to physical and mental health, and they can both be valuable spiritual practices.[2] This evening, when you lie down to go to sleep, try whispering a prayer into the quiet darkness. This may feel strange if this is a new practice for you, but just give it a try and see what questions or hopes emerge from the depths of your heart. You may or may not consider yourself religious, or even spiritual, but we all have something within that is looking for meaning. Prayer, however you choose to do it, could help you find and connect with that meaning.

Intuition:

YOUR CIRCADIAN RHYTHM

Your *circadian rhythm* is the internal rhythm of your body, orchestrated by genes in the suprachiasmatic nucleus located in the hypothalamus in your brain. It is the source of intuition about when to wake up and when to go to sleep, when to eat and when to stop eating, and more. In particular, your circadian rhythm also sends intuitive signals to your body to respond to light and dark, cues your digestive system to eat or fast, governs the release of melatonin and cortisol to make you sleepy or wake you up, and much more. Operating in tune with this circadian rhythm will increase your intuition about how to live well. To take advantage of these circadian cues, try sleeping, waking, and eating consistently most of the time, according to your body's signals. This will train you to detect and respect your natural rhythms so you can get enough sleep and wake up refreshed and rejuvenated, eat natural foods at regular times, and honor your own energy fluctuations. Turn inward to feel and follow these messages, and your intuition will strengthen.

Intuition:
TRACK YOUR SLEEP QUALITY

If you like sleep-tracking devices, they can be useful tools in gauging sleep length and quality, but you don't need them to figure out what kinds of things you are doing that contribute to a good or poor night's sleep. All you need to do is use your attention and intuition. I suggest starting a sleep journal. Tonight, write down what time you turn off the light to go to sleep. In the morning, write down when you wake up, how you *think* you slept, whether you woke up a lot during the night or not, and anything else you remember about your sleep. Then, notice how you feel, even before you get out of bed. Are you rested and alert or groggy and heavy? Next, list all the things you did yesterday that you have an inkling could have led to how you feel this morning. Were you stressed? Did you exercise? Did you eat well, or poorly, or late in the evening? Ponder the previous day for clues and write down what you think were the contributing factors. Do this for a week, then look back for patterns. Do you seem to get better or worse sleep when you do certain things? That's valuable information, and your intuition at work.

Balance:

REM SLEEP

A balanced sleep includes appropriate amounts of REM sleep. REM sleep is the period of sleep in which you do most of your dreaming, so people sometimes call it dream sleep. This is a psychologically and cognitively important sleep stage that helps you learn and remember things better. During REM sleep, researchers believe you process what has happened to you that day, consolidate and store memories, and maybe even work through problems.[3] REM sleep is also essential for emotional regulation, restoring a sense of optimism, and creativity.

Most adults spend about 25 percent of their sleep time in REM sleep.[4] When you don't get enough, some research suggests you will eat more the next day.[5] Caffeine and alcohol consumption in the second half of the day may also interfere with REM sleep.[6] For the best-quality REM sleep, eat a nourishing dinner that's not too high in sugar or fat, don't have any caffeine after noon or alcohol after dinner (no alcohol at all is even better), get seven to nine hours of sleep on most nights, and try to maintain a regular sleep schedule. Institute these healthy sleeping practices and watch the quality of your life improve.

Balance:
DEEP SLEEP

Another critical sleep stage is called *deep sleep*. This is the time when your body does a lot of its repairing, restoration, and perhaps most importantly, flushes waste from the brain, which could improve cognitive function and may even help ward off cognitive decline with age.[7] Deep sleep may also be important for regulating blood sugar and releasing growth hormones for muscle and bone repair.[8] During deep sleep, you experience the longest, slowest brain waves, called *delta waves*, and ideally, the slowest heartbeat and breathing rate. It is the stage of sleep that is hardest to wake up from. Sleep time, and especially deep-sleep time, does seem to decline with age, but adults should ideally spend about 13 to 23 percent of their sleep time in deep sleep.[9] Most people get most of their deep sleep in the first half of the night, so if you stay up too late, you could rob yourself of this vital kind of rest. Regular exercise can also increase time in deep sleep, as this tells your body that you need time to repair and rebuild. Consider an earlier bedtime tonight, and exercising more regularly starting tomorrow, to make sure you have more opportunity for restorative deep sleep.

Rejuvenation:
MAKE YOUR REST LUXURIOUS

One way to wake up looking and feeling fresher is to get your pillows right. Sleeping with your head a little higher than your body will help fluid drain out of your face so you aren't as puffy in the morning. This morning, take a look at your pillows and bedding and consider how you might arrange or improve them to wake up feeling more refreshed tomorrow. Ideally, your body is evenly supported with no bend in your neck. The right pillow cover can also make a big difference. If you want to look the least rumpled, go for silk pillowcases on all your pillows, or at least the one that touches your face and hair. Silk pillowcases will be less likely to leave pillow wrinkles because they stay smooth, and your hair will glide over the surface so you won't wake up as frizzy. An eye mask can also help by blotting out all light, so you get a deeper, more restful sleep. Your sleep quality is integral to your overall health—what better reason to make it a luxurious experience?

Rejuvenation:
HOW'S YOUR SLEEP HYGIENE?

Sleep hygiene—the environment you sleep in and the things you do before sleep—is a huge factor in how well you rest. An important aspect of sleep hygiene is your bedtime routine. Do you have one? When you do the same thing every night, in the same order, preferably at the same time, you send your body cues that it's time to wind down. If you don't have a sleep routine, try instituting one tonight. Turn off all electronics and stop eating at least an hour before bed. Skip the alcohol tonight, if you usually have some. Take a warm shower or bath, which has been proven to increase sleepiness and improve sleep quality.[10] Spend some time reading, journaling, meditating, or praying. Have some romantic time with your partner, or relaxing conversation with family (this is not the time to have arguments). Try to go to bed a little earlier so you can get the deep sleep that tends to happen in the first half of the night—it's important for better brain function and mood. Drift off into your pleasant dreams—then try to do it all again tomorrow! The secret to an effective routine is consistency over time, and it's never too late to get started.

Abundance:

BEAUTIFY YOUR BEDROOM

Another important aspect of good sleep hygiene is to make your bedroom a peaceful haven for sleeping. The ideal sleep environment feels abundantly clean, peaceful, uncluttered, very dark, and around 65 degrees Fahrenheit. It should feel like a sanctuary. Today, take a look around your bedroom. Does it meet these criteria? If not, take a few minutes to pick things up, dust things off, and think about how you might make your bedroom feel more restful, inviting, and abundantly lovely. This doesn't have to be costly. A few basics can make a big difference. Don't use your bedroom as a storage space. Electronics should be moved out of the room. Blackout curtains can help with sleep-disturbing light. And just as importantly, how could you make it more beautiful? New bedding? A fresh coat of paint? Flowers? You deserve a place of rest that feels like a sanctuary. This can be an ongoing project, but it's a fun one and will pay off in sounder and higher quality sleep.

Abundance: STORING
AWAY YOUR ANXIOUS THOUGHTS

If you wake up at night with anxious, racing thoughts, one way to achieve an abundance of calm so you can get back to sleep is to visualize those thoughts as things you can put away temporarily. Imagine the thought—worry about a health issue, finances, relationships, some mistake you made—as a thing outside of yourself, about the size of a beach ball. Picture a large bottomless box with a hinged lid and a lock. In your mind, open the lid of the box. Take that beach ball in your hands, have a look at it, then put it into the box. Close the lid and secure the lock. Imagine there is a blank label on the outside of the box, and a marker next to it. Take the marker and label the box with the category of the thought, like: "Work concerns," "Money worries," "Relationship troubles," "Mistakes." Explore your consciousness for other thoughts you can put away into the correct boxes. When all the thoughts are stowed away, take a few deep breaths and drift off to sleep peacefully, knowing that you can always deal with these issues tomorrow . . . if they still feel like issues, which they may not.

Nurturing:
THE RESTORATIVE POWER OF A NAP

Napping isn't just for toddlers. Research shows that adults who nap can reduce the symptoms of sleep deprivation and may be more creative and productive.[11] The sweet spot for a nap seems to be about twenty minutes. It's not so long that you fall into a deep sleep and wake up groggy, but it's just long enough to get a second wind and feel a boost of energy. Try nurturing yourself today with a quick catnap if you feel tired in the afternoon. Some people are even able to do this at work, which is a workplace improvement I think is long overdue. If you can't nap during the week, a weekend nap can help you make up any sleep debt from the week. Just be sure not to nap too close to bedtime. Wake up by 3:00 p.m. for best results.

Nurturing:
WHAT WORKS BEST FOR *YOU*?

There's a lot of advice about what to do before bed that can lead to better sleep. Some people say not to eat for three hours before bed, while others advise a small snack. Many recommend not exercising at night because it's too stimulating, while others say that gentle exercise like yoga can help you relax and sleep better. But just like other kinds of nurturing, your evening routine is about the way that you feel uniquely cared for. There is no one correct answer for everyone. Figuring out what works best for your personal needs is part intuition and part experimentation. On an evening when you eat late or don't eat, notice how you feel in the morning to determine whether that helped or hurt your sleep. The same goes for exercise. If you work out vigorously after dinner, do you sleep better or worse? Does yoga relax you before bedtime or does it rev you up too much? Tonight, start figuring out what helps you feel most calm and sleepy, so you can tweak your evening routine in ways that will make a real difference for *you*.

Thoughtfulness:
REDIRECT YOUR NEGATIVE FEELINGS

Today, if you are feeling tired, stressed, overworked, or overextended, try channeling that negative energy into something positive by saying at least one thoughtful thing you might not normally say to someone. Then really listen to how they respond. Some ideas:

- "I believe in you."
- "Tell me about what you want most for your future."
- "What's the best thing about your day today?"
- "Is there anything I can do to make your life easier?"
- "I really appreciate the way that you . . ."
- "You're so good at making me feel . . ."
- "One of the things I love the most about you is . . ."

Believe it or not, reaching out to someone else and making them feel good can actually help reenergize you when you are feeling low or exhausted. It's like a coffee break but with much better side effects!

Thoughtfulness:
WHAT YOUR BODY ENDURES

Tonight, give some thought to what your body has had to endure to keep you functioning. Our bodies do the best they can with what we give them, and they have to contend with a lot: incoming toxins from a polluted world, processed food, hours sitting to do work that requires staring at a screen, muscles that don't get enough use, digestion that is taxed and pushed to the limit, the stress of a life that is both too busy and too isolated, and the worry and anxiety related to relationships, work, family, and finances. Our bodies evolved under very different conditions than they now face, and yet they keep our hearts beating, our blood flowing, our lungs breathing, our livers detoxifying, our kidneys filtering, and our brains running the whole show. Everything your body can or can't do today is a reflection of what it has had to endure for you. That's a lot. This evening, have compassion for your hard-working body. It hasn't betrayed you. It has saved you. In this way, you are a walking miracle. So tonight, go to bed early enough that your body can get the rest it needs to recover.

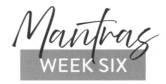

I deserve rest. I deserve a break. When I'm tired or frustrated, I will stop doing and let my body and mind recover.

———————

My sleep is peaceful and deep. Through sleep, I solve my own problems, generate my own energy, and become healthier and more vibrant.

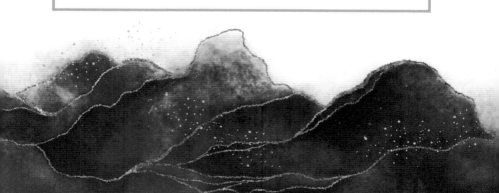

Awaken Your Inner Artist

Creativity comes from trust. Trust your instincts. And never hope more than you work.

RITA MAE BROWN

Voice: WRITING TO REVEAL
WHAT YOU WANT TO SAY

Your voice doesn't just express itself through speech. Writing is another way to express yourself. If you write about what you are thinking, this is a way to "speak" to others (and yourself), but with the advantage of being able to curate and consider your thoughts so they express your meaning more clearly. Whether you keep a journal, write essays about your thoughts and opinions, or compose actual letters to others, writing can reveal threads of thought—and parts of yourself—that you might not have recognized consciously. For some, writing feels difficult, but the more you do it, the more comfortable you will become with this unique form of self-expression. Today, whether you write to yourself or someone else, spend some time putting pen to paper and see what your written words reveal.

Voice : JOURNALING TO UNTANGLE THE PAST

Evening is a good time to journal. Not only can you reflect upon the day, but it's also a quiet and calm way to think about the past. If journaling isn't something you typically do, why not give it a try? If you're having trouble getting started, here's a cue for you: What is the earliest thing you can remember? Your first fond memory? If you aren't sure about your earliest one, write about any memory that comes to mind. (If some of your early memories are difficult, you may not want to write about those at night. Save the more painful memories for when you have energy and time to process.) Think about what you can remember and describe the surroundings—what you saw, what you heard, what you felt. Do you remember particular colors, smells, tastes, or other sensations? Find a moment from your past that feels positive and immerse yourself in it.

Intuition:
JUST LET IT FLOW

Creativity is an excellent way to tap into your intuition. What creative pursuit can you engage in today? Writing, drawing, painting, playing music, singing, dancing, arranging flowers, re-doing a room in your home, even daydreaming can be a creative pursuit. Don't worry about talent or let your critical mind intervene. Just let your creativity flow straight out of your intuition—no editing!—and you may be surprised at the genius results. To get inspired, as you move through the day today, give yourself permission to play. There are no rules. The more you open yourself to your own creativity and let it flow, the more you can get an intuitive sense of what it is you were meant to create as your ideas begin to take shape.

Intuition:
WHAT STIRS YOUR PASSION?

Creativity isn't a talent. It's a choice. It is something you can decide to engage in occasionally, or daily. If you've told yourself you "aren't creative," know that this isn't true. Creativity may come more easily to some people, for many reasons, but it's accessible to anyone. Your intuition can help you discover your inner creativity. What do you love to do? What makes time disappear? You may not exercise your creativity in traditional ways like painting, writing, or playing music. Maybe for you it's how you decorate your home, cook a beautiful meal, or care for your friends. Maybe it's in the way you teach and parent your children, or execute your tasks at work. Those parts of your life that seem to glow when you think about them are the sources for your creative inspiration. Creativity is what adds beauty, interest, and texture to life, and that looks different for everyone.

Balance: SETTING BOUNDARIES
SO YOUR IDEAS CAN FLOURISH

Creativity can be a valuable part of your work, but to feel more balanced, it's useful to make space for creativity that has nothing to do with your profession or usual responsibilities. It can be hard to draw those boundaries, but one way to do that is to shut off all media interaction during times when you want to work on something creative. Distraction is the enemy of creation, so if you really want time to foster your creativity, turn off your phone and block all access to email, texting, and social media. We so seldom get the chance to spend intentional quiet time with our imaginations that doing so can feel foreign at first, but try it a few times and you may be amazed at what your brain can come up with when you eliminate distractions. Find a balance between connection and disengagement with the world, and your creative instincts will blossom.

Balance:
CREATING SPACE

Reflect on how you used your time today and write down—from the moment you woke up to now—how you spent each hour. Where was the free time, when you weren't doing something you had to be doing? Ask yourself: *Did I spend this time in a way that was fulfilling to my soul?* Under the weight of all our responsibilities, we can often either feel pressured to dedicate every waking hour of the day to something that's "productive" or find ourselves drawn toward empty distractions just to give our tired brains a break. On the other hand, when we do engage in the vital and healthful outlet of creativity, we might feel pangs of guilt for indulging in something our fast-paced modern world deems unnecessary. Take another look at the written account of your day. What blocks of time could you have prioritized differently so your schedule feels more balanced between must-dos and want-to-dos, with less precious time wasted? Now, map out your intended schedule for tomorrow, and reserve space for your creative endeavors. There are, after all, only a certain number of hours in the day, and you are the only person who gets to decide what to do with yours.

Rejuvenation:
BECOME A STUDENT AGAIN

How do you rejuvenate a brain that's so often on autopilot? Try learning something new, which is a great way to spark creativity. If your schedule and resources permit, you could sign up for an online class or a continuing education course at a local college. But even learning something small and seemingly insignificant—a new fact or a new technique for executing a daily task—can do wonders to wake up a tired brain. Get curious about someone you know really well and seek to discover something new about them, or find an opportunity to have a conversation with someone you've never met before. Learn the name of a new bird or flower or tree. Learn how to cook a recipe you've never tried, or how to say a sentence in another language. It's not so much what you learn as it is the learning process itself that is so rejuvenating to the emotions and mood, awakening curiosity and a fresh appreciation for everyday things. Learning also rejuvenates the brain, as neural connections form with every new thing you learn, improving cognition and enhancing creativity.

Rejuvenation:
WHAT DO YOU ASPIRE TO LEARN?

Take some time to make a list of all the things you'd like to learn throughout the rest of your life. There is nothing too insignificant or insurmountable, and it's never too late to approach aspirations you've held in the quiet places of your heart. As you make your list, ask yourself why you want to learn it, and how you think you might be different if you learn it. Learning new things may help to head off brain aging, but it can also create a rejuvenated sense of possibility and even a feeling of youthfulness. Imagine that your life experience is a huge, beautiful mosaic. Each thing you learn is a new jewel, stone, or piece of colorful tile that adds to that mosaic. The more you add, the more complex, beautiful, and inspiring that mosaic becomes. Keep learning, and you will make your life a magnificent piece of art that you build upon with each new day.

Abundance: INVEST THIRTY MINUTES A DAY IN YOUR DREAMS

If you spend just thirty minutes each day on something that fuels your passion and makes you feel alive, you'll generate abundant creative energy. This could be something as simple as learning how to play the guitar or something more complex like working on the business plan for that great nonprofit concept you came up with, drawing up plans for your dream home, or finally starting that book you've always wanted to write. Will it be difficult at times? Probably, but allotting thirty minutes each day toward this endeavor will pay off richly in a stimulated intellect and improved overall quality of life. What you do regularly is more impactful than what you do sporadically. Just thirty daily minutes can do more for your progress than spending hours on something once or twice a month. Whatever you dedicate this time to, it should be something you don't normally prioritize. With just thirty minutes a day, your daydreams could become your reality.

Abundance: DO YOU
FEEL STUCK IN A CREATIVE RUT?

Even if you know you want to make more time for creative endeavors in your days, you may still feel creatively blocked. This can happen when you get in a creative rut, and sometimes the best way to get out of that slump is to approach some part of your usual routine in a novel way. Tonight, how could you shake up your routine to get that creative energy flowing again? This could be as simple as changing up your usual dinner or taking a different route on your evening walk. Anything you do that is out of the ordinary for you can be effective. Just find some small way to break from your status quo. You may find that forcing your brain to change up your daily routine can open the door to an abundance of creativity, just by forcing your brain to go off autopilot.

Nurturing:
NATURE'S CREATIVE INSPIRATION

One of the most inspiring ways to nurture your own creativity is to get out into nature. Get your eyes off screens and take in the wondrous masterpiece that is the natural world. Nature is endlessly creative, and just being in nature can help you to feel more creative. People often come up with their most creative ideas while walking through the woods. Today, spend some time outdoors. Whether that means you go for a walk in a local park on your lunch hour or enjoy a long early-morning hike, focus on being present and noticing the details of your surroundings. Take in the varying colors of plant life, wonder at the way the sunlight streams down and hits the grass, listen to the sounds of chirping birds or rustling wind, and feel the cool breeze against your skin. Rather than listening to music or thinking about work, try to focus fully and mindfully on the natural world around you and let this practice relax your body and brain. When you get back to the tasks of your day, allow this lingering sense of unhurried peace to remain with you and inspire you in your creative endeavors.

Nurturing:
LET MUSIC MOVE YOU

Just as our creative spirits are nurtured by nature when we remove distraction and really connect with it, music has comforted, enlivened, relaxed, excited, calmed, and stirred the passions for tens of thousands of years. Music often acts as background noise for our leisure activities or busy days, but what if you took time to simply *be* with an extraordinary piece of music? Try putting away distractions and give a song a chance to inspire and move you. Take some time this evening to sit quietly, with headphones or earbuds if you have them, and listen to some of your favorite pieces of music without interruption. Enjoy a cup of herbal tea or your favorite relaxing drink, put your feet up, and get comfortable. Close your eyes and let the sound fully occupy your consciousness. Where will it take you? This is an incredibly relaxing way to feel nurtured and inspired to create.

Thoughtfulness:
PAY IT FORWARD

Have you ever purposefully "paid it forward"? This is a creative play on the idea of paying someone back. When someone does something nice for you, you pay it forward by doing something nice for someone else. The next time someone offers you a kindness, pass the favor along: If someone holds the door for you, you hold the door for the person behind you. If someone gives you a compliment, you offer praise to another person. But you don't have to wait for someone else's kindness to inform your own. Get creative! Send unsolicited notes of appreciation. Drop off a hot meal or a home-baked dessert to a neighbor. Take donations to the local food bank or supplies to an animal shelter. Pay for a stranger's meal in a restaurant or for someone's coffee behind you in line. These little acts can brighten your day as much as someone else's and give you that reassuring feeling that people remain kind—yourself included! How can you pay it forward today?

Thoughtfulness:
GET INSPIRED BY OTHER CREATORS

You can expand your own creativity by thoughtfully considering the creativity of others. Tonight, spend some time looking at inspiring art, reading beautifully crafted prose or poetry, browsing photos of interior designs or architectural marvels, exploring gourmet recipes in a cookbook, or listening to classical music. Do a bit of research on the creators—who they were and what motivated them. Let this exploration open your mind to the full appreciation of what creativity can manifest and how it can add beauty and a sense of wonder to life.

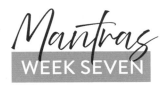

Mantras
WEEK SEVEN

I am a wellspring of creativity,
and I use my gift to add wonder
and beauty to the world.

———————

I marvel at the miracle that is life, and
I participate fully and mindfully each
day with reverence and gratitude.

Warm to Hearth and Home

Ah! There is nothing like staying at home for real comfort.

JANE AUSTEN

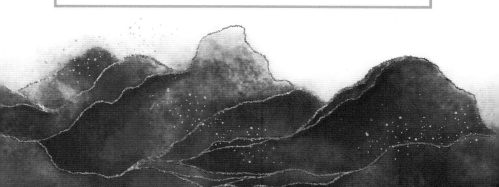

Voice: WHERE DO YOUR LOVED ONES GATHER?

Every home has a room or an area where people tend to congregate. Think about where people like to chat in your home. It might be in the kitchen or dining room, or maybe it's the living room or back porch. Wherever that room is, give it some special attention today. The area where people gather is the heart of the home and the most conducive to the connection that happens through conversation. That space deserves some TLC. Declutter, clean, or add some decor you love to that area of your home. Can you make it even more inviting with a lovely scented candle or cozy throw pillows? Find ways to make this room feel like an even more comfortable space for your loved ones to share and connect with one another.

Voice: YOU ARE THE HEART OF YOUR HOME

This evening, spend some time alone in that part of your house where people come together. Sit still and quiet in that space that might usually be filled with noise. Does it feel different from other parts of your home? Look around and think about what makes *this* particular area the heart of your home, and you may realize that it's actually *you*. Is it the area where *you* prepare food for others? Where *you* ask the family to gather for a meal? Where *you* like to relax, and others are drawn to share in that relaxation with you? Where *you* like to get people talking, interacting, and having fun? A person, much more than a room, is the real heart of a home. Take a moment to revel in all the warmth and love that you offer to the people who gather here.

Intuition:

WHERE DO YOU FEEL BEST?

What is *your* favorite room in the house? Whether it's for socializing or alone time, which part of your house makes you feel the most calm and peaceful? If you aren't sure, use your intuitive sense. Walk around your home, into all the different spaces, and pay attention to how your body responds. Where do you feel tight or tense? Where does your body relax? Where do you feel the most content? Once you've figured out your favorite spot according to your intuitive reactions, think about why. Do you feel best in the kitchen because you love cooking or food? Do you feel best in the study because you love the work you do in that space? Maybe it's the family room because you are happiest when everyone is together. Or perhaps it's the bathroom, where you care for yourself and your personal hygiene, or your bed, where you can't wait to curl up. Give some thought to what it is about your personality that makes a certain room feel best.

Intuition:
CULTIVATE THE AMBIENCE YOU DESIRE

This evening, go to your favorite spot in the house, which you may have just identified this morning. Think about how you spend your time there, and then see if you can do something to make that space even more functional for whatever purpose you use it. What is the ambience of that space? Do you love it because it's relaxing, stimulating, or romantic? Is it a place to learn things or to be creative? See if you can specifically target that feeling and increase it with what you add to—or remove from—that space. Whether it's adding music, flowers, a bookshelf, writing or drawing supplies, or just getting rid of everything *not* related to the ambience you want, a little time spent here can greatly increase your enjoyment of your favorite spot.

Balance: AN EXTERIOR
PRELUDE TO INTERIOR BEAUTY

Do the inside and outside of your home feel balanced? Whether you live in a big house or a tiny studio apartment, how the outside of your home looks influences how you feel when you enter it. Are there things to consider about the exterior of your home that you have control over and that might make your home feel even more inviting? Something as simple as a pot of flowers by the entryway, a welcoming doormat, or a fresh coat of paint on the front door can make a huge difference. Brush those cobwebs away from the exterior lighting, sweep the area right in front of your entryway, and wipe down the door every week or so as part of your regular cleaning routine, and you'll be surprised how different it feels to enter your home.

Balance:

SPEND A LITTLE TIME OUTSIDE

You probably spend more time inside your home than immediately outside your home. To feel a little more balanced at home, especially if you've been inside a lot more than usual lately, try spending some time outside your home, on your own property. Stroll outside in the morning to get some fresh air and sunlight. Step outside in the evening to feel the cooling air or stargaze. If you have a yard, a back patio, or access to a front stoop of a shared building, you could change things up by taking dinner outside and dining alfresco. The outside of your home is your home too. Why not get to know it a little better?

Rejuvenation:
TURN YOUR BATHROOM INTO A SPA

If any room in your house is made for rejuvenation, it's the bathroom. This is the place for practicing personal hygiene, bathing, beautifying, and rejuvenating the body, mind, and spirit. You may rush in and out of your bathroom a few times a day, but what if that room was a little more like a spa? Display your most reliable skin-care products on a mirrored tray, accompanied by a scented candle or humidity-loving plants (ferns love a steamy room). Give your mirror a squeaky-clean scrub, lay out some freshly laundered towels, and fill a bath basket with decadent soaps, body wash, or essential oils that will make your next bath or shower feel like a truly rejuvenating experience. These small details combine to give your bathroom a vibe that will make you want to pamper yourself daily.

Rejuvenation: THE TREATMENT YOUR BODY DESERVES

Treat your time in the bathroom tonight as a chance to intentionally rest and unwind from the day. If you are able, play relaxing music and take more time than you usually do to wash your face and hair, brush your teeth, and scrub your nails with care. Try accompanying your usual skin-care routine with an exfoliation treatment, vitamin C serum, or soothing mask. Give your hair a moisturizing treatment, try dry brushing on your arms and legs, then relax in bathwater scented with lavender essential oil. Mindfully engage in these activities and think about how you are combatting the aging effects of modern life with self-care, good hygiene, hydrotherapy, aromatherapy, and the care and nourishment that your precious skin deserves.

Abundance: WHERE DO YOU DEAL WITH FINANCES?

Today, think about the part of your house where you pay bills or handle money. This might also be where you do the tasks involved with your profession or household management. It could be a whole home office, a desk tucked away in the kitchen, or another room where you keep all the important paperwork for your family. How well-ordered do you keep this space? Do you rush through financial chores because they make you uncomfortable, or do you relish the task of getting organized, paying bills, and balancing budgets? Today, see if you can clean up and organize to make this space more efficient and more pleasant. Respecting how money comes in and out of your life can help you overcome anxieties about it as you become more consciously aware of, and by extension in better control of, your finances.

Abundance: A HARMONIOUS FLOW OF RESOURCES

Tonight, think about how resources flow in and out of your life. There's money, of course, but there are also other resources like the material things you own, the food you eat, the hospitality you offer to others, the friendships you invest in, and the quality time you spend with family. Do these things feel rightly ordered? Are you overly focused on any one resource more than the others? You create an atmosphere of abundance when your home is a place where all of these resources work in tandem. Do you focus equally on what you bring in and what you send out? Think about how you might make this flow of energy—because resources really all boil down to energy—happen more smoothly, with incoming resources unblocked and outgoing resources appropriately let go of. Imagine your life is like a bridge over a river. Resources constantly flow in and constantly flow out, but beneath the bridge, there is always an abundance of river.

Nurturing:
MAKE THE BEDROOM A SANCTUARY

The bedroom is surely the most nurturing room in the house. It's a place for all kinds of care: romantic connection with a partner, relaxation and restoration on your own, or reading stories to children and tucking them into bed. The bedroom should be a sacred space where you feel completely comfortable, at ease, and safe. Earlier, we talked about how to create a sanctuary for rest in your own bedroom, but what about the other bedrooms in your home? Do they feel welcome, private, safe, and comforting? Think about how you could make these spaces feel even more secure and comfortable for those who sleep in them, whether adults, children, house guests, or even pets. You could remove items that don't add to the ambience of comfort and security (like electronics, things stored in bedrooms that don't really belong there, or just general clutter), and add a few new touches that make the bedroom feel like a refuge. More comfortable bedding, a soft rug underfoot, bedside books, a beautiful water glass, shuttered or curtained windows, and soft lighting can all improve the ambience of a room and create a more nurturing space.

Nurturing: INTENTIONALLY CARE FOR SOMEONE THIS EVENING

Do the people in your home typically retreat to their own separate spaces to relax in the evenings? This evening, try staying in a shared space and spending some extra time nurturing someone in your household. That might mean turning off the television and spending some quiet one-on-one time with your partner to really talk to each other in a loving and supportive way. Turn in at the same time tonight—especially if you don't usually do that—and share some physical intimacy, even if it's just a loving touch or a goodnight kiss before you both fall asleep. Another option is to spend extra time putting children to bed tonight. Pamper them a little—focus on brushing teeth, brushing hair, and getting clean. Help them put on their comfiest sleepwear. Read an extra book before bed and cuddle with them and make them feel seen, safe, and loved. Or let yourself be the recipient of your own nurturing tonight. Put fresh sheets on your bed and have a cup of chamomile tea. Put on your nicest pajamas. Light a scented candle, play some soft music, and curl up with a good book or write in your journal. You could even give yourself a hug before you drift off peacefully.

Thoughtfulness:
BE A GOOD NEIGHBOR

Do you know your neighbors? Many people don't know the people who live nearby or may only know them in passing. But when everyone in a neighborhood keeps an eye out for one another's safety and well-being, it adds to everyone's sense of security. Remember that we used to rely on one another for survival. We still have that instinct. We also know isolation can lead to sickness, heart disease, cognitive decline, and depression, and that a wider social circle contributes to greater happiness and health.[12] Is there a thoughtful act of service that you could offer a neighbor who might need assistance, like raking their leaves, shoveling snow, or taking care of any in-home maintenance such as changing air filters or light bulbs? Could you give a friendly wave, or say hello and pause for a brief chat when you see someone passing by (if it seems appropriate)? You don't have to be friends with everyone who lives nearby, but by being a good neighbor, you can help others to feel less isolated.

Thoughtfulness:
INVEST IN YOUR NEIGHBORHOOD

Spend some time this evening thinking about your neighborhood. Are there ways you might be able to help make it a better place? Make a list of some things you might do to make your neighborhood a more pleasant and welcoming place to live. If you're the outgoing type, you might organize a group to clean up litter or a neighborhood block party for socializing, or you might just suggest an informal meetup with neighbors to chat over coffee or tea so you can all get to know each other a bit better. If you prefer to keep to yourself, walk around your neighborhood more often to get a sense of what's going on and how well people are doing. Do you notice any safety issues? An area where cars go too fast? Someone who lives alone or who is elderly or infirm? Could you be a safe point of contact for kids walking home from school each afternoon? There are many ways to improve your neighborhood and foster an environment of security and friendliness.

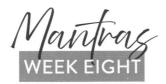

Mantras
WEEK EIGHT

My home is my refuge. It
protects me and shelters me,
and I care for it in return.

There's no place like home.

Feel the Earth Beneath Your Feet

*Those who contemplate the beauty
of the earth find reserves of strength
that will endure as long as life lasts.*

RACHEL CARSON

Voice:

LET NATURE SPEAK

Nature has a voice, but it can be difficult to hear, especially if you never listen. There are profound benefits to spending more time focused on the natural world around you, including lowered stress, lowered blood pressure, increased levels of "happy" neurotransmitters like endorphins and dopamine, less depression and anxiety, and a greater sense of inner calm.[13] To really hear the clarifying and guiding voice of nature, take some time to step outside today—head to your own backyard, a local park, a walking trail in a nearby natural area, wildlife refuge, or forest—and prepare to simply listen. Take a few minutes to sit down, relax, and breathe. Then, close your eyes and focus on the sounds around you. What do you hear? Birds, trees, wind, leaves, waves? Spend about ten minutes just listening. You aren't waiting to hear actual words. Just let nature speak to you, and notice what feelings arise. After you've connected with the natural world through listening, you might as well get up and go for a walk. Exercising in nature is therapeutic, too!

Voice: HOW DOES LISTENING TO NATURE AFFECT YOU?

How did your day go, after spending a little time listening to nature's voice? Did you feel differently than you do on days when you spend all your hours cooped up indoors? Were you calmer? More clear-headed? Did you have an easier time making a decision or focusing on your work? Think about what was different, if anything, then spend some time writing about it, if you feel so moved. If you didn't notice any difference, do you need a higher nature "dose"? Maybe more regular time in nature is exactly what you need. Nature exposure is good medicine, and "taking" that medicine consistently will likely make the positive effects more obvious.

Intuition:

INSTINCT VERSUS INTUITION

People often confuse instinct and intuition. They aren't the same, but they are related. *Instinct* is something we often think about in terms of nature. How do birds know their migration patterns? How does a gazelle sense that a lion is hunting it? Through instinct. This is based in safety and survival, and people have it too. We're born with it. It's a feeling that spurs action without premeditated thought, like when you decide not to walk down a particular street because you have a bad feeling about it, or you sense a thunderstorm coming. *Intuition* is more advanced. It's an inner knowing that is informed by instinct but also by experience, wisdom, and mindfulness. Intuition is something you can improve on because it is based on observation and experience. Today, think about the differences between instinct and intuition, and see if you can sense both of them at work within you.

Intuition:
NATURE IS A GREAT TEACHER

Did you come to any interesting conclusions today as you thought about instinct and intuition? If you aren't sure about how these are working within you or whether you have access to either, have faith that you can become more attuned to your natural instincts, and you can train and develop your intuition. Nature is a great teacher in both capacities. Instinct is a precursor to intuition, so start there. When you are out in nature, tune in to your responses and try to sense the energies and interactions in the natural world. If you're on a walking trail, do dark shadows and rough foliage warn you against turning down a particular path? If you're out for a beachside stroll, would a chill in the air and increased strength of the tide tell you of an incoming storm? This can awaken your instincts, which may be buried under the habits of a modern life spent indoors and overconnected to technology. Intuition, on the other hand, comes from a state of calm mindfulness, during which you take in subtle information about how the world works. As you spend time in nature, pay close attention to everything around you rather than distracting yourself. Bank that information in your subconscious mind. Sensing uncovers instinct. Mindful observation tunes intuition. Nature can connect you to both.

Balance: THE EXTRAORDINARY MIRACLE OF MORNING

Some people like to wake up to watch the sunrise and greet the day, while others prefer the peaceful calm of a sunset. I admit I'm more of a sunset person, but once in a while, I wake up in time to catch the sunrise, and I find it awe-inspiring. While sleeping on a schedule—going to bed and waking up at about the same time every day—is a healthful habit, when it comes to an appreciation of nature, sometimes it's nice to see the world performing wonders you don't usually get to witness. If you tend to sleep past sunrise (most people do), try getting up a little bit earlier now and then to experience how the dark of night gives way to morning's light. The air smells especially fresh, the birds sing with the most cheer, dew sparkles on the ground, and as the sun rises, it puts on a most extraordinary light show. If you didn't wake up in time this morning, how about tomorrow?

Balance: LET EVENING'S DARKNESS ENVELOP YOU

This evening, take a walk as the sun sets and experience what it's like to see and feel the night taking hold around you. Most people spend their evenings in front of screens these days, but there's an incredible performance happening right outside your front door every single evening. When it's cloudy, you may not get the same sunset drama you could get on more interesting weather days. Even so, being outside as the world grows dark and all the parts of nature that come awake at night begin to stir can be a spiritual experience. Being outside during both sunrise and sunset—a dose of nature at both ends of the day—can also help calibrate your circadian rhythm so you sleep better and feel more balanced overall. Remember, humans used to live outside all the time, so we are built to see and experience the natural cycles of light and dark. Just as a sunrise can stir your soul awake, letting yourself get wrapped up in the darkness of an oncoming evening can lull you into peace and rest.

Rejuvenation:

TAKE A WALK AMONG THE TREES

Have you heard of the practice of *forest bathing*? That's a modern term for a concept that is far from new: walking among trees. Forest bathing—or *shinrin-yoku* as it's known in Japan where the technique was first systematized and popularized—is a form of ecotherapy. It's easy to do: simply take a walk through an area with a lot of trees. Trees emit aromatics, such as essential oils released by evergreen trees, which may increase the body's production of the white blood cells that support the immune system,[14] which could help your body get better at fighting infections and may also reduce inflammation. Forest bathing also appears to lower blood pressure and stress, as well as reduce depression and anxiety.[15] This may be because the body instinctually recognizes its natural environment, and the body responds in kind. While much of this is theoretical or anecdotal, there is no doubt in my mind that walking through forests is good for the body, mind, and soul. Can you take an hour out of your schedule today to spend some time in a tree-filled area? Give it a try and see if it makes everything feel a little bit better.

Rejuvenation:
HOW TO STAY GROUNDED

Grounding, or earthing, is a practice of connecting—quite literally—with the earth. Many believe that grounding causes physical changes in the body, like lowering blood pressure, respiration rate, and heart rate; reducing inflammation and stress-hormone production; and improving blood flow, sleep, and energy.[16] This is a simple technique: connecting your bare skin to the earth. You could do this by walking barefoot in the grass or on a beach, or sitting or lying on the ground. The theory is that when the body meets the earth, the electrical charge of the planet flows into the body, causing these positive changes. Although mainstream medicine isn't on board yet, there is some research showing the benefits of this practice,[17] and I believe that any connection to nature will have positive physical and/or mental health effects, since we evolved for millions of years living outside most of the time and have now become so separate from the natural world. So get back to your roots, slip out of your shoes, and get grounded.

Abundance:
GROW TO GIVE

While we often think of abundance in terms of acquiring, which may mean taking from something else to have more for ourselves, abundance in the natural world is about generosity and fantastic diversity. Trees and plants generate oxygen and fill the soil with nutrients, even as they use nutrients. Then they return to the soil to add all their nutrients back in, to feed even more abundant life. When something becomes overabundant, something else comes in to use it, like an insect infestation drawing wildlife to a new source of food. Just look around to see the ebb and flow of nature's abundance, as every part of an ecosystem works in harmony. Nature, in its season, may be abundantly rich with snow and ice, rain and mud, lush and dormant plant life, rich and regenerating soil. There are insects and sea life, birds and mammals, grasslands and deserts and oceans and forests, with each system generating resources that lead to the abundance of other resources. Nature doesn't take to grow. It grows to give. Spend some time reflecting on this wonder and think about how you can apply this practice to your own life. In what areas might you, like nature, be able to grow in order to give?

Abundance: WHERE DO YOU HAVE MORE THAN YOU NEED?

What are *your* natural resources? Think about what you are abundant in right now. Whatever it is—energy, time, creativity, financial means, compassion—think of yourself as part of nature. Nature generates abundance and shares it with others, making everyone more abundant, and then that abundance comes back to its source. Are there ways you could replicate this? You can be like those trees that send out water, nutrients, and chemical messages through their root systems and fine networks of fungi that connect all the trees in a forest. This giving nourishes and encourages the growth and flourishing of other trees. This morning you reflected on areas in which you could grow more in order to give more, but what about the resources that you already have in abundance? How can your own surplus be shared in order to help others become more abundant? When you do this, you may find that abundance flows easily back to you. You may not always get the same thing you gave, but you might get something infinitely more valuable to you: self-esteem, purpose, opportunity, happiness.

Nurturing:
PRACTICE WITH PLANTS

Nurturing a plant is much different than nurturing a person or even an animal, but if you are new to nurturing, a plant is a great place to start. Plants have simple but specific needs and require regular attention. If you can keep a plant alive and flourishing, you've mastered Nurturing 101. But even if you have other things to nurture (a partner, children, pets), taking care of a plant can cross-train your nurturing skills. Consider bringing a plant into your home, learning everything you can about how to care for that particular plant, then seeing how well you can make it grow. One budget-friendly way to do this is to visit a garden store or big-box store and look for clearance plants that are in need of a rescue. These may cost only a few dollars, or even less. See if you can take them in and bring them back to health.

Nurturing:
GRADUATE TO A GARDEN

If you can keep a plant alive and healthy, the next step might be to try gardening. This healthful and gratifying hobby can connect you with nature in a whole new way. You could start a garden in your own yard, or in pots on a patio, or get a space in a community garden. Whether you want to add more beauty to your life and the world through a flower or ornamental-plant garden, or produce food by growing a vegetable garden, you can nurture nature to achieve your gardening goals. Tend and nurture your plants and pay attention so you notice when they need something. Not every plant will survive in every climate, and it can take some trial and error to figure out what level of commitment you can give and what ultimately works for you. This is all part of the learning process. Gardening is good exercise, well worth the effort, and it could become a new passion to enrich your life.

Thoughtfulness:
GIVE THE GIFT OF NATURE

We've talked a lot about how you can personally reap the benefits of connecting with nature, but how about sharing nature's gifts with others? Try doing at least one of these things this week:

- Gift a basket of fruit or homegrown vegetables to someone who may have a difficult time getting to the grocery store.
- Take a friend on a walk through a natural area you've discovered or want to explore.
- Pick a few wildflowers, then press and frame them as a gift. Note where they came from and the date.
- Gather friends and visit a local farmer's market or an independently owned vegetable, fruit, or flower stand.
- Add touches of nature to each family bedroom: potted plants, seashells in a glass bowl, collections of beautiful rocks, or vials of sand from different beaches.

Thoughtfulness:
YOUR NATURAL CONNECTIONS

This evening, spend some time meditating on your relationship with nature throughout your life. Think about specific times when you interacted with nature as a child. What is your earliest memory of the outdoors? Was nature a refuge, or did it seem foreign? Did your family spend time together in nature, or did you like to go explore by yourself? What are your best memories of times in nature? Do you have memories of nature being frightening or intimidating? Or was it your favorite way to escape or engage in childhood fantasies and play? How has nature shaped your personality, even if it's just in some small way?

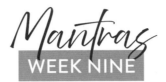

Mantras
WEEK NINE

I move with the rhythms
of the natural world.

———————————

Nature is my teacher.

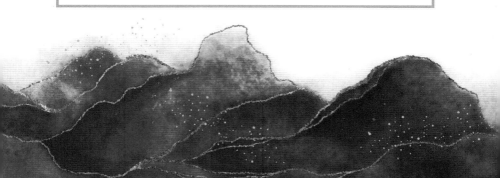

Engage in the Art of Conversation

Once a human being has arrived on this earth, communication is the largest single factor determining what kinds of relationships he makes with others and what happens to him in the world about him.

VIRGINIA SATIR

Voice: CONSIDER HOW YOUR WORDS WILL BE HEARD

There is a difference between what you say to someone and what they hear. Sometimes we mean one thing, but the person we're talking to hears something completely different. This can feel incredibly frustrating. You may think they *should* have taken you at your word, or understood what you meant, but nobody can control how someone else interprets what you say. When having a conversation, especially about a sensitive issue, take a moment before you speak to contemplate your intended message. How would it sound from the other person's point of view? How would you feel if someone said to you what you're about to say? This one small step—of considering how your words will be heard, not just how you will say them—can make you a more empathetic and thoughtful conversationalist, and could very well sidestep hurt feelings, misunderstandings, or escalating arguments.

Voice: FUEL YOUR
WORDS WITH PURPOSE

As you look back over the day, think about how you used your words. Were there things you said that you regretted, either immediately after or later? Things that came across differently than you intended? Things you hesitated to share, but were glad when you did? What could you have said differently in situations that didn't go the way you hoped they would? Were there opportunities to speak that you didn't take? Times when you wished you would have said nothing at all? Take an inventory of how accurately, truthfully, compassionately, and bravely you used your voice today. Tomorrow, maintain this same mindfulness as you move throughout the day and practice articulating *exactly* what you mean to say.

Intuition: FOCUS OUTWARD AND THE RIGHT WORDS WILL COME TO YOU

Some people habitually think out loud without any discernment or forethought about what they intend to say. Others go over their words internally and incessantly, ruminating on how they should express themselves, sometimes so much so that they never say anything at all. But there is middle ground between these two extremes. Your intuition can guide your words. This may be the most effective way to communicate with others because it takes into account other people's body language, expressions, inflections, and energy. This can lead to words that are more compassionate, purposeful, and meaningful to the other person. When your focus is turned toward another person and you let your intuition flow, the right words are much more likely to spring forth. After all, it's a conversation, not a performance. Try this today. When you are talking with someone, focus all your attention on them. You don't have to analyze what you see. Just take it in, then speak from the heart without overthinking it.

Intuition:
SPEAK THROUGH SILENCE

Intuitive communication doesn't always require words. Sometimes a touch, or even a look, says more than spoken words ever could. Tonight, experiment with intuitive nonverbal communication. Let your intuition guide you about what communication might be more powerful than talking. Consider what you know and feel about the person you are with. Do they need a hug? A gentle touch? A smile? Do they just need someone to listen with compassion while they get something off their chest? When you talk with them, try backing away from language and see what happens. Does this method of communication make you feel closer or strengthen your bond with that person?

Balance: BE AN ACTIVE
LISTENER AND A SELF-AWARE SPEAKER

Real communication is a balance between talking and listening. Some people tend to be talkers. Rather than listening, they wait to talk again. Others are great at listening but have a hard time getting their words in. Either way, being only a talker or a listener is likely to lead to imbalanced communication and missed connections. To balance your conversations, try these tips:

- When someone else is talking, resist the urge to focus on what you want to say next. Instead, look them in the eye and really try to listen to what they are saying.
- Be aware of how long you've been talking. Are you getting too detailed? Are you talking about things other people don't necessarily want or need to hear about?
- Try not to interrupt while the other person is speaking.
- Actively listen to what the other person is saying for details you can build on to move the conversation forward.
- Respond thoughtfully to what the other person says before expressing your own ideas.

Balance: HOW WAS YOUR CONVERSATION QUALITY TODAY?

Think back over the day and replay some of the conversations you shared with other people. Do they feel balanced? Could you have listened better? Were you unable to express your opinion? Did you say how you really felt, or did you mask it to avoid conflict? Were you compassionate and thoughtful in your responses? Communication is difficult and it takes practice, so don't berate yourself for doing something you believe you could have done better. An awareness of where imbalances are happening in your own communication style is a way to learn how to communicate better.

Rejuvenation:
PERSONALIZE THE CONVERSATION

Even though it barely scratches the surface of meaning, small talk can be absolutely exhausting. It's an easy way to fill an uncomfortable silence or pass the time, but it does little to feed the hearts or minds of the people engaged in it. Rather than simply going along with vapid small talk that will leave you feeling drained, why not personalize the conversations you have today? Try to find ways to use superficial conversation topics as springboards to discussions rooted in unique or shared experiences that will leave both you and the other person feeling energized and rejuvenated. If someone comments on the weather (a typical small-talk staple), ask them what their ideal climate is. What's their favorite thing about the current season? Do they prefer the coziness of the winter season or the freedom of summertime? You might even get them talking about a special memory that they hold dear from this time of year. People are endlessly complex, so rather than dreading the boredom of small talk, try approaching others with genuine curiosity and watch as an interesting conversation unfolds.

Rejuvenation: OFFER THE GIFT OF YOUR ATTENTION TO OTHERS

Think back to one of the personalized conversations that you had today. Your curiosity coupled with the little bit of extra effort it took to ask interesting questions likely created an opportunity to connect with someone you might have otherwise overlooked. When we engage in communication styles that aim to fill others up, as opposed to just passing the time, our focused attention becomes a rejuvenating gift that lifts spirits and awakens minds. Think about some of the people you're likely to cross paths with tomorrow, such as the barista at your favorite coffee shop, the cashier at the grocery store, or even someone in your household. How can you engage that person with intentional curiosity?

Abundance: SPEAK SO THAT PEOPLE WANT TO LISTEN

Some people have a hard time making themselves heard, but you can learn how to speak so that other people are more likely to listen to you. Here are some ways that can make you feel more abundantly heard:

- Look people directly in the eyes when talking to them.
- Keep your voice steady and project—don't mumble or whisper.
- Get to the point. If you want to express something, come out and say it. Be direct.
- Keep it short. Let the conversation go back and forth.
- Look for nonverbal cues of waning attention in others, such as wandering eyes or glances at their phones. Stop talking and regroup.
- It's okay to say things like, "Now this part is important," or "I really need you to hear what I'm about to say."
- Listen well to others, and they may be more likely to listen well to you.

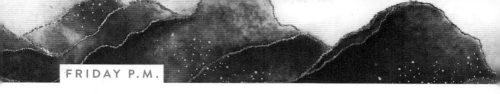

Abundance:
DID YOU FEEL HEARD TODAY?

Reflect on the day and how well you feel you were heard. Whether your attempts at making sure your words registered with others were successful or not, think about those exchanges. Are there things you could have done differently? Is the person you are trying to talk to simply not emotionally available or able to listen for reasons of their own that have nothing to do with you? Some people just aren't very good listeners, and that's not your fault or responsibility. Whatever the case, let go of the stress or obsessive thoughts you have about what you wish would have happened, and repeat this affirmation to yourself as you sit quietly and breathe: *My words matter. What I think is important. How I feel is real.* Even if someone else didn't listen very well to you today, you can take some time to listen attentively to your own feelings.

Nurturing: COMMUNICATE
WITH YOUR INNER PAIN

If you find yourself feeling a little low, it may be because you are carrying too heavy of an emotional burden. One way to nurture your emotions is to forgive yourself for something. This is a profound act of self-compassion and internal communication with your emotional pain. Sometimes we don't even realize the emotional loads we are carrying, so we don't understand why we feel so sad or heavy, but you can lighten your load a bit. Think of something you feel guilty or regretful about, then make a list of things you could do to make it right. Could you apologize to someone? Do something to help someone? Admit that you were wrong? Fulfill a promise you made? Or would your most powerful action be to truly, deeply forgive yourself for a mistake you made or a wrong you committed, so you can finally move forward again? The relief and feeling of lightness after you do this can be profound.

Nurturing: FORGIVENESS
SETS YOU FREE

Are you carrying the weight of emotional wounds inflicted by others? Forgiveness does not erase the past, but it is a way to nurture yourself by setting *yourself* free from the agony of being chained to a painful history. Forgiveness cannot depend on something someone else does, because then they continue to have control over you. Forgiveness has to come from within *you* and you alone, regardless of how the other person feels. To begin the process, have an imaginary conversation with the person you have chosen to forgive. This is a conversation that never has to happen with the real person. What matters is your own experience. Express how you feel. Tell them what they did to hurt you. Then practice saying to them, in your own mind: *I forgive you and release you. I am letting go of this pain.* This can be an intense experience (and a therapist can help with this), but when you are ready, you may find that it sets you free.

Thoughtfulness:
PROPER CORRESPONDENCE

In a world of emails and texts and social media posts, an actual handwritten letter can be a poignant and thoughtful way to show appreciation for someone. Think of someone whom you truly appreciate. Instead of sending a digital message, take some time to sit down and write to someone who holds a meaningful place in your life. Yes, with an actual pen on actual paper, or on a card. Express how you feel about that person. Be specific and sincere. Let them know how grateful you are to know them, and tell them exactly why. What did they do for you? What do they mean to you? What will you never forget about them? Whether this letter is to someone you haven't seen for a long time or to someone you see every day, the mere act of communicating this way is a tribute to someone's importance in your life. And unlike a text or an email, it might be something they keep and cherish for years to come.

Thoughtfulness: SAY WHAT YOU DIDN'T GET THE CHANCE TO BEFORE

Are there words that have remained unsaid to someone who is now gone from your life? When someone leaves, moves away, or passes away, a common regret is not getting to say what you wanted to say to them. It may be too late to say those things to that person directly, but you can still express them. This evening, sit quietly and think about that person, then imagine they are sitting in front of you. What do you want to say? Speak the words, or write them down. Say everything you never got to say. Just communicating it—hearing the words you speak or reading what you wrote—can release a lot of pain and help you to feel more resolved about the loss of someone you care about. Get those words out of your head, and plant them in your heart, where they can blossom.

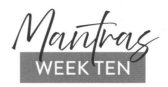

Mantras
WEEK TEN

I speak with clarity and I tell my truth.

———————

I listen with compassion to the words—
and to the meaning behind the words.

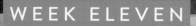

Indulge in Sensory Wisdom

For ourselves, who are ordinary men and women, let us return thanks to Nature for her bounty by using every one of the senses she has given us.

VIRGINIA WOOLF

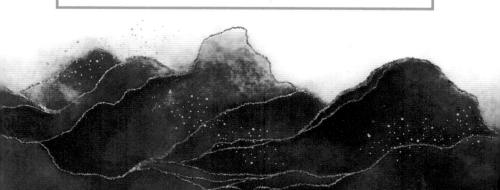

Voice:

WHAT IS A BODY SCAN?

A *body scan* is a meditative practice that focuses on minute sensations in the physical body, which can be clues to discover where you need to focus extra attention. It's a way to purposefully tune in to your body's voice and how it's trying to communicate with you. It's also relaxing and can help you calm down if you tend to wake up with nervous energy aimed at the day ahead. To try it, lie on your back on a flat surface, like a yoga mat on the floor or a firm bed, using pillows to make you feel comfortable. Take a few deep, slow breaths, then focus on your toes. Wiggle them. Feel them. Notice any sensations, pleasant or uncomfortable: pain, itching, soreness, ease. Then move to your feet and notice any sensations. Slowly move up your body, pausing on each part: calves, knees, thighs, hips, belly, heart, chest, shoulders, upper arms, elbows, lower arms, hands, fingers, throat, neck, chin, mouth, cheeks, nose, eyes, ears, forehead, scalp, and finally, the crown of your head. Try to feel every sensation, from the obvious to the subtle, then see if you can feel your whole body at once. What is it trying to tell you? What does it need from you?

Voice : LET GO AND REPEAT

A REFRAIN OF GRATITUDE

This evening, take a few moments to sit quietly and imagine every weight you have carried on your shoulders today—every difficulty, obligation, compromise, sacrifice, mistake, or tough conversation—slowly lifting off your shoulders. Feel the lightness of letting go. Let a sense of ease permeate your body. Relax your shoulders. Unfurrow your brow. Let that weight float slowly up, then imagine it dissolving into thousands of tiny white stars that flicker and go out in the night sky. Feel yourself floating with the freedom and peace of existing solely and completely in this present moment. Now, say this aloud three times: "I release these things, and I greet this moment with gratitude."

Intuition: EXPLORE THE EMOTIONS TIED TO SCENT

Aromas may be among the strongest of triggers, bringing back memories and strong feelings even when we don't consciously register the connection. You can further refine your "scents" of intuition with practice. Today, notice all the aromas and odors you can perceive, both pleasant and unpleasant. Purposefully use your sense of smell throughout the day to detect the aromas of food, flowers and other plants, people, different rooms within buildings and in your home, or the smell of clothing, bedding, and linens. Try closing your eyes to remove visual distractions and home in more intensely on this important sense. Which aromas make you feel peaceful, joyful, and calm? The more you become aware of the effects that particular scents have on your state of being, the more you can intuitively seek them out to cheer you up or calm you down.

Intuition : SEND SCENT
SIGNALS TO YOUR BRAIN AND BODY

Aromas can bring back memories, but you can also link specific aromas to certain actions, to help shape your own subconscious reactions in the future. One nice way to do this is to learn to associate a certain scent with bedtime as part of an evening ritual. Just as the scent of coffee can make you feel more alert in the morning, certain scents—such as lavender, sweet orange, cedarwood, jasmine, and vanilla—can help induce a relaxed feeling. Ideally, choose a scent that doesn't already have an emotional association but that you enjoy and that feels relaxing to you. Whether in your soap or bodywash, moisturizer, or even a lovely scented candle, try folding one of these scents into your evening routine. Do this regularly, and you'll begin to associate that scent with calm, winding down, and sleepiness, which can help you get a better night's rest.

Balance:

BE THE SILENCE YOU SEEK

We live in an increasingly loud world. In addition to the actual noise of daily life—traffic and chatter and machinery—our lives are bombarded with digital noise. The cacophony of calls, emails, messages, news notifications, and social media can leave us feeling like there's no place where we can just escape into silence. Today, try balancing out the incessant noise of the physical and digital worlds by actually embodying the quietness you seek. You don't have to take a vow of silence, but what about a one-day vow of being silent-ish? Apply focused effort to staying as quiet as possible today so you can become hyperaware of the noise around you—how much of it you take in and how it affects you. Throughout the day, notice what kinds of noises accompany your life that you aren't usually aware of. Most importantly, use this day of quiet to evaluate what kind of digital noise you can eliminate—or at least limit—so that you emerge from your period of self-imposed silence to engage with noise in a more balanced way.

Balance: THE DAY'S NOISE
TURNS INTO EVENING'S SONG

If you're still engaged in the practice of silence we instituted this morning, this evening presents an opportunity to evaluate noise in a very different way than you did during the daylight hours. If you like to hike or walk outdoors, you're probably used to hearing the sounds of daytime, but depending on your environment, those noises can change dramatically after the sun goes down. Step outside this evening and take a moment to listen to the sounds of the night. Whether you are in a big city, a small town, or a natural setting, notice how the sound profile changes. Think about how early humans lived, and hearken back to a time when technology didn't drown out the natural noise of the world. In the dark, they couldn't rely on their vision like they could during the day, so survival was often largely based on what they could hear. You can recapture this valuable human instrument that we once depended on for safety cues. Imagine you are relying only on sound as you listen to the night. What is it telling you? Be quiet, be still, and listen. What song is the evening singing?

Rejuvenation: THE REVIVING POWER OF ESSENTIAL OILS

Essential oils can wake you up, energize you, rejuvenate your mind, and boost your mood, all through your sense of smell. Even if you aren't very sensitive to scents, essential oils are powerful enough to have a rejuvenating effect on just about anyone. To energize yourself or simply feel like you've turned the clock back a few years, try any of my favorite rejuvenating essential oils:

- geranium
- frankincense
- orange
- clary sage
- lavender
- rosemary
- ylang-ylang

Put two to three drops in your palms, rub them together, and cup them over your face. Inhale the scent. Take five long, slow breaths and focus on the scent impressions and how they make you feel.

Rejuvenation:
BEAUTY BREATHING

To relax, feel calmer, and be more in tune with your senses and the mindful experience of the present moment, there is no more powerful practice than focusing on your breath. Conscious breathing is a meditative practice to rejuvenate the mind, but beauty breathing is one of my favorite practices for a quick boost in mood and appearance. This simple exercise can melt away those worry lines and make you look fresher and happier in just five minutes. To me at least, a calm and happy face is a beautiful face. Here's how to do it:

1. Set a timer for five minutes.
2. Inhale slowly and as fully as possible to a slow count of four (or about four seconds).
3. Hold your breath for a slow count of five (or about five seconds).
4. Exhale slowly and as fully as possible for a slow count of eight (or about eight seconds).
5. Hold your breath after the exhale for a slow count of two (or about two seconds).
6. Repeat until the five minutes are up.

Abundance:

A WORLD ALIVE WITH COLOR

Of all our sensory cues, visual information comes to us most abundantly, but we take much of that visual information for granted. Imagine that your world was black and white until this very moment, and now—it's in Technicolor. Today, tune in to what you see as you move through this vibrant world. Notice colors, textures, tones, and levels of light and darkness. Look for subtle things you might not normally notice. Let yourself feel an appreciation for the beauty in the colors, textures, and patterns of all things ordinary, subtle, and seemingly inconsequential. This practice can bring a whole new dimension of mindfulness into your life and help you to appreciate how amazing and impactful it is to *see*.

Abundance:
EATING AS AN EXPERIENCE

What feels more abundant than luscious tastes? Today, pay attention to your fifth sense every time you eat or drink. Do you taste salt, sweet, sour, bitter, or savory (sometimes called *umami*)? Pay extra attention to the texture of the food. Really dig in to the sensations of taste—identify what you enjoy, what you don't, and why—to help you refine your palate. Get a clearer sense of what you truly enjoy and what you don't really like. Focusing mindfully on taste helps with the kind of intuitive eating we discussed earlier, but it can also help you to get more enjoyment and a deeper satisfaction from food. Eating is, after all, one of life's greatest sensory pleasures.

Nurturing:
HOW DOES THAT FEEL?

Of all the senses, surely touch is the most nurturing. As you move through your day, pay attention to as many touch sensations as you can, from inanimate objects you feel with your hands—the cold metal of a stair railing or the warmth of a full coffee cup—to the touch of another person if they shake your hand, give you a hug, kiss you goodbye, or just tap your arm to emphasize a point. How do those sensations make you feel? Notice the touch of your clothes on your body, the shoes on your feet, the breeze or sun on your skin. We are exquisitely sensitive to touch, but people don't normally notice or they would be so distracted that they wouldn't get anything done! Let yourself get at least a *little bit* distracted today, as you focus on what emotions come up as you consciously touch different items and connect physically with people and whether they feel grounding, nurturing, or something else.

Nurturing:
THE GIFT OF YOUR TOUCH

This evening, think about how the sensation of your physical touch can be nurturing to other people. Make an effort to connect physically to your loved ones this evening. This can be as simple as a hug, the squeeze of a hand, or an impromptu back rub if someone is feeling stressed. You might rock a baby, cuddle a child, or be intimate with your romantic partner. Whatever you do, be mindful of the sensation of touch in particular. Notice how the other person responds in order to gauge whether your actions are having a nurturing effect. You might learn something valuable about what kind of touch gets the most welcome response from someone you love.

Thoughtfulness:
NAVIGATING SENSORY SENSITIVITY

Different people are extra-sensitive to different sense impressions. For some people, bright lights might be too intense. Others may be sensitive to loud noises. Some may have an acute sense of smell and be easily offended by strong odors. Others may be averse to strong tastes. Some people are acutely sensitive to touch and may not want to be touched at all without knowing it's coming and consenting. If you know, or find out, that someone has a sensory sensitivity, be thoughtful about how you interact. That may mean turning down the lights, lowering your voice, adjusting what you are cooking, or not going in for that hug. Rather than being offended if someone says, for example, "You're talking so loud!" the most thoughtful reaction is to be empathetic and adjust. If you're the one with a sensitivity, a polite way to let others know is to be honest but kind. You might say something like, "You may not know this, but I'm really sensitive to bright lights. Do you mind if we go somewhere with less harsh lighting?" Either way, you'll be thoughtfully engaging with other people in a way that can help everyone feel more comfortable and secure.

Thoughtfulness : HAS OVEREXPOSURE DULLED YOUR SENSES?

Did you know that overexposure to certain sensory stimuli can be stressful? You may not realize at first that you have a sensitivity, but exposure may be stressing you out. If you frequently experience loud noises, bright lights, strong smells or tastes, or unwanted touching, and you don't say anything, these experiences could be a source of chronic stress you didn't realize was affecting you. Take some time this evening to think about how you react to sensory impressions. What do you love to see and what do you find unpleasant? Are there sounds that feel calming, like music or falling rain, and sounds you realize you really dislike, such as traffic noise, machinery, or crowd noise? Are you very sensitive to smells, or do they have little effect on you? Are you a super-taster, who has a strong reaction to particular flavors, or can you eat just about anything with no problem? Are you a hugger, or someone who dreads being embraced? Understanding your own sensitivities is a thoughtful way to understand yourself better. Figuring out how to minimize exposure to stressful sense impressions could be good for your physical and mental health.

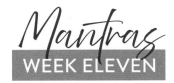

I use my five senses to understand
the world and live mindfully.

———————————

I experience my senses reverently
and with sensitivity.

Thrive in Your Nine-to-Five

To find joy in work is to discover the fountain of youth.

PEARL S. BUCK

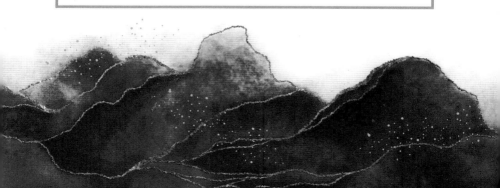

Voice:

SPEAK UP

Are you afraid to be big, bold, and opinionated? Whether you are working to be acknowledged in your career, trying to make your thoughts heard at a social gathering, establishing ground rules with someone in your life, or just attempting to ease some of your stress, how assertively you express yourself can make all the difference. Sometimes, being big and bold is what you may have to be if you need to stand up for yourself and act authentically, rather than how everyone else thinks you should act. Some people have the idea that women are supposed to have soft voices and defer; perhaps this is one reason why the word *bossy* seems usually to be reserved for girls and women. But this old-fashioned notion doesn't serve anyone. If you feel you've been silenced in some way, is it time for you to take up some space? When you feel ready, step out of the shadows and speak up for yourself and others courteously but firmly and clearly. You aren't being bossy. You are being *a boss* who isn't afraid to turn up the volume. The world can benefit from your unique brilliance, and don't let anyone tell you otherwise.

Voice:

GET OUT OF YOUR HEAD

Perseveration, or rumination, is to think about something repeatedly to the point where it becomes unproductive and stressful. There's a fine line between productive thought and ineffective overthinking. Sometimes what you really need is to talk to someone else. Whether you're navigating an issue in your work environment, untangling a financial worry, mending a tough family rift, or just escaping a cycle of self-criticism, getting out of your head and using your physical voice can really help. Sometimes just telling a friend about your problem out loud can help you to see the solution. An objective person (this could be a counselor) might see the situation in a much less convoluted or problematic way and could help you reframe. If you've been obsessing about something, see what happens if you voice your concerns to someone. You might be surprised that what seemed like an insurmountable problem is actually easily solved.

Intuition:
WHAT FEELS RIGHT?

Sometimes you really do have the answers within, but the way to unearth them isn't about thinking harder. When you are facing a big decision, like how to handle a dilemma at work or whether to take a new job, it's always a good idea to weigh all the facts and consider the pros and cons. However, intuition can also help, especially when two paths seem even in terms of the objective facts. There is so much information in your subconscious mind that can inform your decisions, that it doesn't make sense *not* to consult your intuition. Today, when you need to make a choice, even a small one, take a time-out, close your eyes, and ask your inner self: *What feels right?* Then, without trying to answer, stay very quiet and just listen. Oftentimes, within a few minutes and sometimes right away, the answer rises to your conscious mind. The more you do this, the easier it gets, and it's a great way to feel more confident about your decisions.

Intuition:

DECODING YOUR DREAMS

Dreams are one way the subconscious mind works out problems. While many dreams seem random, some may have important messages for you about what direction to take or can shed light on your feelings about something you are contending with. Keeping a dream journal can help you to remember your dreams and also to look back on them to figure out what they might mean. The memory of a dream disappears quickly after waking, so keep a notebook and a pen next to your bed. As soon as you awaken, jot down as much as you can remember—words, images, feelings. Go back at the end of each week and look over what you wrote. Even if your dreams seemed random in the moment, the meanings might be much clearer in retrospect. In any case, dreams can at least prove to you how creative and amazing your brain is!

Balance: WHAT IS WORK-LIFE BALANCE, ANYWAY?

You probably hear a lot about work-life balance, but I've come to understand that such perfection isn't very realistic. Nobody can ever completely balance work and life. And what does that mean, anyway? Isn't work part of your life? I think what people mean when they talk about work-life balance is that it's important not to let your *entire* life become about work. It can be very easy to overidentify with work to an extent that you may allow it to determine your self-worth, or you may find yourself prioritizing work over your personal relationships, in practice if not in theory. Today, take some time to contemplate how you balance your work with all the other parts of your life. How do you allocate your attention and energy on a typical day? You may discover that you aren't always putting your attention where you want it to be. Now that you see it, can you begin to shift it?

Balance: HOW DO YOU PRIORITIZE YOUR TIME?

As you continue observing your work-life balance, you may find that the relative time you spend on different parts of your life doesn't reflect your priorities. Say, for example, that your family is your top priority, but in actuality, you typically spend more time at work than at home. Is your life organized to reflect what matters most to you? Many are surprised to find the answer is no. Of course, for many jobs, you have to be in a physical work space for a certain number of hours, but what about all the additional hours you spend thinking about unfinished tasks, answering emails or phone calls after hours, or just doing "one more quick thing"? To get your priorities clear, make a list of all the things you spend time on, with categories such as work, family, romance, friends, leisure, travel, hobbies, passion projects, creativity, and philanthropy. Put them in order according to what matters most to you (be honest—nobody has to see it), then assess how the time you actually spend in each category reflects your priorities. How could you make some adjustments to feel more balanced?

Rejuvenation: SAY NO, DELEGATE, AND STAY IN YOUR LANE

How do you rejuvenate when you've got too much work, too many responsibilities, and too much stress? Step one is to create some boundaries. Here are some boundary-setting strategies to restore your energy:

- Learn how to say no. How many unnecessary things do you agree to simply because your default is to say yes? Unless you actually *want* to do it, say no. Practice saying it in front of the mirror. "No, I'm sorry, but I simply don't have the bandwidth for that right now." Be firm.
- Delegate. If you take on too much, it's 100 percent okay to ask for help. No one can do it all. Let others contribute.
- Stay in your lane. If you tend to take on everyone else's problems or responsibilities, start handing those things back to their original owners. (That includes children, as long as those responsibilities are age-appropriate.)

Rejuvenation : YOUR RELATIONSHIP WITH BOUNDARIES

If you have trouble with boundaries, spend some quiet time considering why this is. Do you want to feel needed? Is it hard for you to see someone else struggling? Do you compare yourself to others you think are contributing more than you are? Is it possible that you've become a workaholic, or addicted to a high-stress lifestyle? Do you think you don't deserve, or don't get to have, any time for yourself? Really think about this and explore the reasons. This can be incredibly enlightening and give you new insight into how you might be contributing unnecessarily to your own stress. You might not be able to change everything at once, but making even small moves to establish firmer boundaries can be energizing and rejuvenate your energy.

Abundance:
THE ART OF DOING NOTHING

In this fast-paced world that so highly values work and achievement, one thing people increasingly lack is patience. It's hard to be patient when the world expects instantaneous answers, quick action, and 24/7 access. As such, the vital virtue of patience is becoming a lost art. Things used to move much more slowly, and that's not always a bad thing. Attention spans have shortened, and many can't last more than a few minutes without checking their smart phones. If you want to become more abundant in patience, try practicing *niksen*, which is the Dutch concept of doing nothing. Try doing this for five minutes today. Sit outside or in a favorite spot in your home, set a timer, and just simply . . . be. It may seem excruciating at first, but when you intentionally repeat this practice over several days, you may find yourself feeling less of a need to seek distractions at other points during the day as well. Whether in line at the supermarket or in a waiting room before an appointment, set aside the phone, and you might realize that engaging your senses and actually focusing on where you are in the moment becomes more enjoyable than random scrolling.

Abundance:
PATIENCE AS A PRACTICE

This evening, continue the patience practice that you began this morning, but this time, think of it as a restorative act to increase your patience abundance. Set a timer for ten minutes and do absolutely nothing to engage your mind other than existing exactly where you are. Feel free to play instrumental music or ambient noise, but stay away from any and all screens. Close your eyes, take deep breaths, and let the past hours of the day fade away. Your brain will begin to calm down and learn that sometimes, it's okay to just relax into the now. Eventually you can increase the time you spend on your patience practice. Can you work up to fifteen minutes? Maybe even thirty? If you can, you'll feel like a patience master! This will greatly increase your patience and likely will help you become a calmer, more mindful, and in many cases a more productive person.

Nurturing: DAYS OFF ARE NECESSITIES, NOT LUXURIES

Weekdays may be all about the rush of work and responsibilities, but you deserve to dedicate the weekend to nurturing. Nurture yourself and others with outdoor time, family gatherings, getting together with friends, or alone time to restore the energy the week drained from your body and mind. Spend some time on activities that make you feel pampered and relaxed or creative and inspired. It's important to take at least one or preferably two days off from work every week. It's not a luxury. It's a necessity if you want to manage your stress and get or stay healthy. And isn't Saturday the perfect day for it? What can you do to turn off your work brain and nurture yourself today?

Nurturing: HONOR THE PROMISES YOU MAKE TO YOURSELF

Were you able to truly take the day off today? If not, was this unavoidable, or did you get persuaded to do something you didn't really have to do? Think about how you could prioritize your downtime more effectively or with more assertiveness. You don't owe anybody an apology or an explanation. It's fine to say, "Unfortunately, I'm not able to do that today." But if you like, you can always add, "I have family plans today," or "I have a previous commitment," or, "I wish I could, but today doesn't work." Of course, sometimes work does feel nurturing and enjoyable, and if that's the case and you want to say yes, that can be just as beneficial for your stress. Did you do something that felt nurturing and enjoyable today? If not, make a plan for next Saturday, and stick to it! Promise yourself.

Thoughtfulness : YOU CAN ONLY CONTROL HOW YOU REACT

The most stressful part of work can be other people, especially when dealing with conflict. Even though you have no control over what others say or do, you may still find that their actions have a huge impact on your own sense of contentment in your work life. When someone disappoints or frustrates you, it's important to remind yourself that all you can control is how you react. One way to do this is to reframe how you think about what someone else said or did. You may think you know what drives them, but part of living a more thoughtful life is to make allowances for what you do not or cannot know. You can't know what drives someone else's behavior. You would have to know everything about them—their entire past and all their experiences—to understand why they act the way they do. But what you can know is that whatever they are saying or doing, even if it's supposedly about you, it's probably not really about you. All you can do is communicate with honesty about how you can both move forward, then release yourself from the conflict. Sometimes it's hard not to react with anger or hurt, but if you can separate what others do and say from how you feel about yourself, you can greatly improve workplace relations . . . and life itself.

Thoughtfulness:
OFFER THE BENEFIT OF THE DOUBT

This evening, practice reframing an unpleasant interaction with someone. Think back over the past work week, to when someone was rude, got angry, or said something unkind to you that stung. Consider what that person might have been going through that could have impacted how they treated you. Perhaps they just received some bad news. Maybe they are having personal problems or issues at home. Maybe they are recovering from a traumatic event. Instead of holding on to residual anger or hurt from the situation, let your thoughtfulness guide you to give that person the benefit of the doubt. When people stoop to hurtful words or actions, it's usually coming from a place of deep hurt within themselves. Putting your own feelings aside and contemplating what they might be going through can help you embrace sympathy and understanding, which makes it so much easier to release yourself from anger and avoid saying something that will only escalate the situation. This can help you let it go, now and in future scenarios when this happens again (and it will).

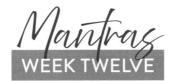

I move effortlessly between times of work and times of rest, times of joy and times of sadness, times of achievement and times of failure, times of excitement and times of peace, times of expectation and times of disappointment, times of love and times of loss, knowing that everything happens in its own time.

I can't control other people. I can only control my reactions to other people. I let the rest go.

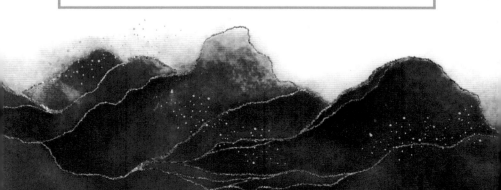

Follow Your Passions and Find Your Purpose

The way to achieve a difficult thing was to set it in motion.

KATE O'BRIEN

Voice: JUST A DREAM, OR YOUR POTENTIAL REALITY?

Do you have a hidden dream? A quiet hope or ambition you've kept to yourself? Something you don't dare tell anyone for fear that voicing it or taking it seriously will guarantee it won't ever come true? But what if your dream could become your reality? If there is something you really want to achieve in your life—travel to a foreign country, start a small business, move to a new city, buy a home—even if it sounds impossible, the first step in potentially reaching your goal is to determine how much you actually want it. So, *say it out loud*. Get used to saying it. How does it sound when you say, "My dream is to . . ."? How does it sound when you say it in the mirror? Try it out on a friend. Words are the way to begin to manifest a dream, or to help you realize it's not something you actually want as much as you thought. Try it today. Give voice to your dream and begin to explore whether or not it could actually come true.

Voice:

START MAKING PLANS

This evening, think some more about your dream. We all have fantasies, and that's fun. But if voicing your dream creates a yearning in you, and you realize this is truly your goal, your passion, something you desperately want to do in your life, then why not start making a plan? This evening, begin a list of action items. Start small with three steps you can take to move in the direction of your dream. Could you open a savings account? Research travel options to visit your dream destination? Enroll in an online course to learn a language? Even if you later change your mind and life takes you on another path before the dream is fully realized, you will have learned something about yourself. Or maybe these steps will be the beginning of a great adventure in which all your dreams really do come true. How will you know if you never give it a shot? Whether or not it all happens the way you imagine, you will know you gave it a shot. And . . . what if it does?

Intuition:
WHAT MATTERS TO YOU?

Each one of us has a purpose in this life. Some people are quite sure about their mission, but many people struggle to define what this is. Your intuition can help you to begin understanding your unique gifts and desires, which can help you clarify your purpose. Sit quietly and take a few deep breaths to calm and clear your mind. Then, simply ask yourself: *What matters to me?* Don't try to answer with your conscious mind. Just sit quietly and listen. Feel what rises out of your subconscious. If nothing comes on the first try, repeat this once or twice a day. Even if nothing concrete comes up, you might start to get ideas and inspirations that could lead in the right direction. It's about focus. Deep down inside, you know what it is. Getting quiet and using your intuition can help you unearth why you are here.

Intuition : LET YOUR PASSIONS POINT TO YOUR PURPOSE

Passion and purpose aren't always the same thing, but they can be. To help you discover your purpose, look to what you most love to do. What gets you deeply excited? What has always interested you, maybe even since childhood? What makes you want to get out of bed in the morning? If the answer eludes you, start noticing what you really love to do. Your passions can be clues to your purpose. Maybe your purpose is to bring more beauty into the world with your artistic talents, to nourish others with good food, to learn more about different cultures through travel, or to teach others how to take good care of their bodies. Maybe you are a healer, a hero, a visionary, or an inspiration. Whatever it is, don't stress if it takes you a while to find it. Just know that you *are* here for a reason, and that you'll know what that reason is when the time is right.

Balance: MAKE TIME
FOR WHAT YOU LOVE TO DO

You can truly love to do something and still prioritize everything else ahead of it. But why not prioritize what matters so much to you? Pursuing your passion can reduce stress and measurably improve your quality of life, so it's vital that you intentionally make space for that thing you *love* to do, that drives you, that makes you feel so alive. You may feel pressured to be productive all day, every day, but pursuing that thing that gives your life its vibrancy *is* productive because it fills your cup, so you've got more resources to get your other tasks done and help others. Today, carve out some time to do what you *really* enjoy, whatever it is. Put it on your calendar and treat it like an unbreakable appointment, as important as any meeting or responsibility.

Balance: HOW DID YOU SPEND EACH HOUR?

How did you spend your time today? Were you successful at making some time for your passion? If so, how did that impact the rest of your day? If not, why did you prioritize other things? Give some thought to how your day went, then write down how you spent each hour, like you might write down a budget. Look it over and circle those times that look to you, on paper, like wasted time. How could you have used that time to do something that brings you joy? You'll never get a do-over on today, but think about how you could spend tomorrow's precious hours in a more balanced way, which includes things that really matter to you and bring you joy.

Rejuvenation:
GIVERS MUST ALSO RECEIVE

Many people feel a call to serve or help others and know that this is their purpose in this life. But what if your purpose is draining you? This is actually quite common. Service jobs like nursing, teaching, and caregiving can be highly stressful, and people in these professions are prone to burnout. But other jobs that aren't so obviously service-oriented can also involve demands that come at the expense of your own health. Parents of young children often experience this. Even when you know you are making a difference, it's easy to overextend. If you are a giver, it's important to take care of yourself at the same time. Give as much to yourself as you give to others. This is incredibly difficult for some people, who feel compelled to give but have a hard time receiving. Yet, if you don't replenish your energy, you'll have nothing left to offer. Make sure you take *at least* one full day off every week, if at all possible, and spend some of that day doing something just for you and nobody else. If you want to fulfill your purpose, this is an absolute requirement. Doctor's orders!

Rejuvenation:
YOU ARE PART OF THE WHOLE

Tonight, try this meditation. Sit or lie down comfortably and take some long, slow, deep breaths. When you feel relaxed, imagine stepping outside of yourself. See yourself sitting or lying there, eyes closed, breathing. Now slowly zoom out. Imagine you are moving to the doorway and seeing yourself inside that room. Then, zoom out slowly, to the ceiling of the room, above the building, above the entire city. Imagine a golden thread connects the you above to the actual meditating you. Keeping that golden thread intact, zoom out again, to look down on the state, then the country, the continent, and the whole planet. Zoom out even more and see yourself as part of a solar system, a galaxy, and finally, of infinite space. Stay here for a while, as if you are floating in space, that golden thread shimmering, your awareness tied all the way back to you meditating. Now, follow that golden thread all the way back to that room where you began. When you're ready, open your eyes and reflect on the fact that you are part of something unimaginably big, and yet your presence is unimaginably important.

Abundance:
YOU ARE WONDERFULLY MADE

In the midst of life's demands, it's easy to get caught up in feelings of inadequacy. But you are a treasure trove of abundant gifts that enrich the world around you and the people in your life. Are you rich in passion? Passion is essential for a vibrant life. I don't mean romantic passion (although that's nice, too). I mean that deep excitement for something you love to do. Today, make a list of things that make you feel passionate, that you love to do, that matter to you, or that give your life meaning. The longer the list, the better, because to feel passion is to feel alive. It is to know who you are and what you want to do with this life, and that may just be the greatest way to feel truly abundant. No matter what you have, what really matters is who you are and what you can do. Now, make a list of all the things you've done that have contributed something, no matter how small, to other people or to the world, in any way. Go back over your whole life and make this list as long as you can. After you've finished, read back over the list and marvel at how rich you really are. Feel gratitude for all the gifts you've been given and all the good things you've done. The world would be poorer without you.

Abundance:
THE GIFT OF GRATITUDE

This morning, you made a list of the many gifts you offer the world. Tonight, make another list of all the gifts that the world has given to you. Start with the material things that provide comfort to your life: a roof over your head, food to satiate your body, clean water to bathe in and drink. Now, think about the activities that spark your happiness. Does caring for your family bring you great joy? Do you have a fulfilling job? Do you spend time on charitable work or hobbies that make the world feel like a brighter place? Now, most importantly, reflect on your most cherished relationships. Who are the people who hold value and create meaning in your life? Think about what makes each of them special to you. Try to maintain this gratitude in the days ahead so that when you walk in the door of your home, spend time doing something you enjoy, or connect with the people you love, you can—in that very moment—feel grateful for the abundant gifts in your life.

Nurturing:
YOU ARE ENOUGH

You are enough. You lack nothing. You are everything you need to be right now. It's good to evolve, learn, and grow in wisdom and maturity. It's good to have passions and a purpose, meaningful work, and goals for the future. All that is true. But what is also true is that who you are in this moment is enough. You are fully and completely *you*, and that is all you need to be. You don't have to keep looking for some great goal you're going to achieve. You don't have to be any different or any "better" than you are right now. Release yourself from the pressure to do and be more. Some people might say, or imply, that you should change, be different, or do more, but what other people think about you is none of your business. What matters is what *you* think about yourself. Could you be better at certain things? Sure, we all could. If you work at it, you can get better at anything, and if you decide to do that, great. But even so, right now, you are you, and you have everything you need to be yourself. All you have to be is you, and that's enough.

Nurturing:
DO YOU KNOW YOUR CORE VALUES?

While there are some high-level values most people have, around which society has been built, each of us has certain values we consider to be most important. Knowing what your core values are can give you a deep sense of stability, a firmer sense of who you are, and a compass by which to navigate your life. Tonight, take some time to think about the values that are most important to you. Make a list of ten, then narrow it down to three. Put those top three in order of priority. As you make life decisions, work toward your purpose, and engage with your passions, these values can guide you. Here are some examples of core values to consider for your list:

adventure	happiness	knowledge
beauty	harmony	loyalty
creativity	health	peace
family	independence	pleasure
financial security	integrity	romance
freedom	intelligence	security
generosity	kindness	service

Thoughtfulness:

CELEBRATE GROWTH

Today, reflect on who you were when you first started this book and who you are now. How has your life changed? Have you developed new habits, set new goals, or invested in your physical health? Are you more tapped into your senses, in tune with childlike wonder, or connected with nature? Are you sleeping better or feeling more creative? How has your home environment and community involvement changed? Have your new communication skills improved your relationships? Are you practicing your passions and living out your purpose? Think about what you've changed, and honor how far you've come on this journey of life. Never stop growing, but do stop to celebrate your growth every so often. You are an amazing being, and every step you take to make your life more vibrant will make a difference, both for you and for the world that gets to benefit from the great gift that is you. You are a blessing. I hope you always remember that.

Thoughtfulness:
A FOND FAREWELL

This is our last evening together (although you can revisit any step of this journey anytime), so tonight, let's step back and look at the big picture of your life. Imagine your life is a book, a little like this one but much, much longer. Your very own *Book of Life*. Imagine that every day of your life so far is one page. Imagine flipping through that book, from the day you arrived on this planet all the way up to this moment. That story brought you here—all the mundane moments as well as the life-changing moments, and everything in between—to the page that is today. How do you want the rest of your story to go? And how do you want that story to end? There's no way to know how long this book will turn out to be, but one thing's for sure: You are its only author. It's your life. It can be as vibrant and as intentional as you choose. So pick your colors. Choose your images. And start writing the rest of your story today. No matter how it's gone so far, my wish for you is that it will be a story you're glad and grateful you lived—the magnificently authentic, totally unique, captivatingly original story of *you*.

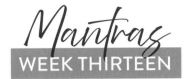

Mantras
WEEK THIRTEEN

I contemplate who I am, what I believe, what my purpose is on this earth, and how I want to live my life. I may not always know the answers, but I will always ask myself the questions.

I am the author of my own *Book of Life*, and only I can decide how my story will go.

Notes

1. Raed Mualem et al., "The Effect of Movement on Cognitive Performance," NIH National Library of Medicine (April 20, 2018), https://www.ncbi.nlm.nih.gov/pmc/articles/PMC5919946/.

2. Sala Horowitz, "Health Benefits of Meditation: What the Newest Research Shows," *Alternative and Complementary Therapies* vol. 16, issue 4, (August 2010): 223–228, http://doi.org/10.1089/act .2010.16402.

3. "Sparse Activity of Hippocampal Adult-Born Neurons During REM Sleep Is Necessary for Memory Consolidation," Nature Index, *Journal: Neuron* (May 20, 2020), https://www.nature.com/nature -index/article/10.1016/j.neuron.2020.05.008.

4. H. R. Colten and B. M. Altevogt, eds., "Sleep Disorders and Sleep Deprivation: An Unmet Public Health Problem," NIH National Library of Medicine (2006), https://www.ncbi.nlm.nih.gov/books /NBK19956/.

5. James A. Horne, "Human REM Sleep: Influence on Feeding Behavior, with Clinical Implications," *Sleep Medicine* vol. 16, no. 8 (August 2015): 910–916, https://doi.org/10.1016/j.sleep.2015.04.002.

6. Soon-Yeob Park et al., "The Effects of Alcohol on Quality of Sleep," NIH National Library of Medicine, *Korean J Fam Med*, 36(6) (November 20, 2015): https://www.ncbi.nlm.nih.gov/pmc/articles /PMC4666864/.

7. Maiken Nedergaard and Steven A. Goldman, "Glymphatic Failure as a Final Common Pathway to Dementia," NIH National Library of Medicine, *Science*, 370(6512) (October 2, 2020): 50–56, https://www.ncbi.nlm.nih.gov/pmc/articles/PMC8186542/.

8. Kristen L. Knutson, "Impact of Sleep and Sleep Loss on Glucose Homeostasis and Appetite Regulation," HIH National Library of Medicine, *Sleep Med Clin* 2(2) (June 2007): 187–197, https://www.ncbi.nlm.nih.gov/pmc/articles/PMC2084401/ and J. R. Davidson et al., "Growth Hormone and Cortisol Secretion in Relation to Sleep and Wakefulness," NIH National Library of Medicine, *J Psychiatry Neurosci* 16(2) (July 1991): 96–102, https://www.ncbi.nlm.nih.gov/pmc/articles/PMC1188300/.

9. H. R. Colten and B. M. Altevogt, eds., "Sleep Disorders and Sleep Deprivation: An Unmet Public Health Problem," NIH National Library of Medicine (National Academies Press, 2006), https://www.ncbi.nlm.nih.gov/books/NBK19956/.

10. Shahab Haghayegh et al., "Before-Bedtime Passive Body Heating by Warm Shower or Bath to Improve Sleep: A Systematic Review and Meta-Analysis," NIH National Library of Medicine, *Sleep Med Rev* 46 (August 2019): 124–135, https://pubmed.ncbi.nlm.nih.gov/31102877/.

11. Jeanne S. Ruggiero and Nancy S. Redeker, "Effects of Napping on Sleepiness and Sleep-Related Performance Deficits in Night-Shift Workers: A Systematic Review," NIH National Library of Medicine, *Biol Res Nurs* 16(2) (April 2014): 134–142, https://www.ncbi.nlm.nih.gov/pmc/articles/PMC4079545/.

12. John T. Cacioppo and Stephanie Cacioppo, "Older Adults Reporting Social Isolation or Loneliness Show Poorer Cognitive Function Four Years Later," BMJ Journals, *Evidence-Based Nursing* vol. 17, no. 2, https://doi.org/10.1136/eb-2013-101379 and Suwen Lin, Louis Faust, and Pablo Robles-Granda et al., "Social Network Structure Is Predictive of Health and Wellness," *Plos One* (June 6, 2019), https://doi.org/10.1371/journal.pone.0217264.

13. Matthew P. White, et al., "Spending at Least 120 Minutes a Week in Nature Is Associated with Good Heath and Wellbeing," Scientific

Reports, June 13, 2019, https://www.nature.com/articles
/s41598-019-44097-3.

14. Qing Li, "Effect of Forest Bathing Trips on Human Immune Function," NIH National Library of Medicine, *Environ Health Prev Med* 15(1) (January 2010): 9–17, https://www.ncbi.nlm.nih.gov /pmc/articles/PMC2793341/.

15. Yuki Ideno et al., "Blood Pressure-Lowering Effect of *Shinrin-yoku* (Forest Bathing): A Systematic Review and Meta-Analysis," NIH National Library of Medicine, *BMC Complement Altern Med* vol. 17 (August 16, 2017): 409, https://www.ncbi.nlm.nih.gov/pmc/articles /PMC5559777/.

16. Howard K. Elkin and Angela Winter, "Grounding Patients with Hypertension Improves Blood Pressure: A Case History Series Study," NIH National Library of Medicine, *Altern Ther Health Med* 24(6) (November 2018): 46–50, https://pubmed.ncbi.nlm.nih .gov/30982019/, and Gaetan Chevalier et al., "Earthing: Health Implications of Reconnecting the Human Body to the Earth's Surface Electrons," NIH Nationsa Library of Medicine, *J Environ Public Health* 291541 (January 12, 2012), https://www.ncbi.nlm.nih .gov/pmc/articles/PMC3265077/ and James L. Oschman et al., "The Effects of Grounding (Earthing) on Inflammation, the Immune Response, Wound Healing, and Prevention and Treatment of Chronic Inflammatory and Autoimmune Diseases," NIH National Library of Medicine, *J Inflamm Res* (2015): 8, 83–96, https://www .ncbi.nlm.nih.gov/pmc/articles/PMC4378297/.

17. James L. Oschman et al., "The Effects of Grounding (Earthing) on Inflammation, the Immune Response, Wound Healing, and Prevention and Treatment of Chronic Inflammatory and Autoimmune Diseases," NIH National Library of Medicine, *J Inflamm Res* 8 (2015): 83–96, https://www.ncbi.nlm.nih.gov/pmc /articles/PMC4378297/.

About the Author

Dr. Stacie Stephenson is a recognized leader in functional medicine focused on integrative, regenerative, and natural medicine modalities. In addition to her functional medicine and anti-aging board certifications, she is a Certified Nutrition Specialist and Doctor of Chiropractic Medicine. Dr. Stephenson is the founder and CEO of a new health and wellness media venture, VibrantDoc, and serves as Chair of Functional Medicine for Cancer Treatment Centers of America (CTCA). She is also the author of the bestselling trade book *Vibrant: A Groundbreaking Program to Get Energized, Own Your Health, and Glow.*

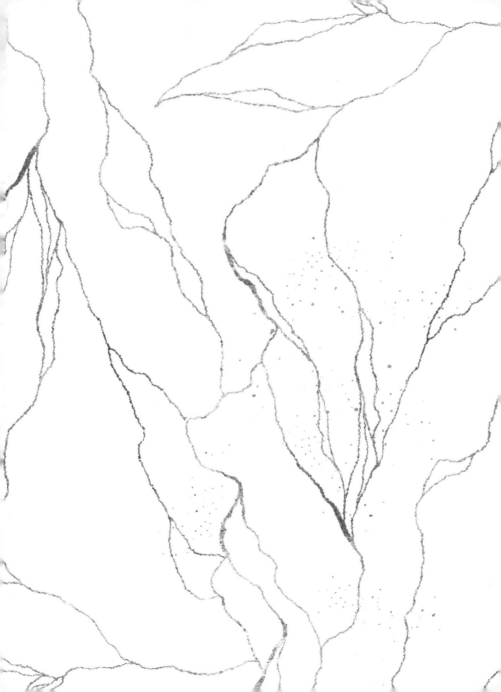

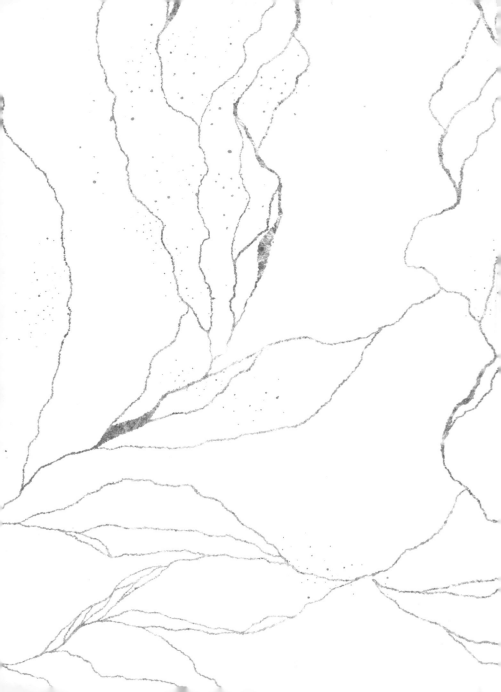